1995

TAKING CARE OF OUR OWN

TAKING CARE OF OUR OWN

A YEAR IN THE LIFE OF A SMALL HOSPITAL

SUSAN GARRETT

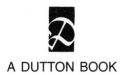

A DUTTON BOOK

DUTTON
Published by the Penguin Group
Penguin Books USA Inc., 375 Hudson Street,
New York, New York 10014, U.S.A.
Penguin Books Ltd, 27 Wrights Lane,
London W8 5TZ, England
Penguin Books Australia Ltd, Ringwood,
Victoria, Australia
Penguin Books Canada Ltd, 10 Alcorn Avenue,
Toronto, Ontario, Canada M4V 3B2
Penguin Books (N.Z.) Ltd, 182–190 Wairau Road,
Auckland 10, New Zealand

Penguin Books Ltd, Registered Offices:
Harmondsworth, Middlesex, England

First published by Dutton, an imprint of Dutton Signet,
a division of Penguin Books USA Inc.
Distributed in Canada by McClelland & Stewart Inc.

First Printing, July, 1994
10 9 8 7 6 5 4 3 2 1

 REGISTERED TRADEMARK—MARCA REGISTRADA

LIBRARY OF CONGRESS CATALOGING-IN-PUBLICATION DATA:
Garrett, Susan
    Taking care of our own : a year in the life of a small hospital / Susan Garrett
        p.   cm.
    ISBN 0-525-93819-2
    1. Rural hospitals—Maine—York. 2. Hospital administrators—Maine—York. I. Title.
RA975.R87G37   1994
362.1'1'0974195—dc20   93-47660
                                                                                CIP

Printed in the United States of America
Set in Sabon
Designed by Leonard Telesca

To my beloved family:

George P., Bill, George G., Alice, David,
Jennifer, Ruth, and Alice Benedict Dunn

and to the memory of Anne Carnicelli

ACKNOWLEDGMENTS

A number of friends and colleagues were more than generous with their good advice during the writing of this book. Grateful thanks to Staige Blackford, Margaret Gromlich, John F. Harlan, Jr., Cynthia Hayes, Edwina Juillet, James Kennan, Matthew J. Lambert, M.D., Linda Mewshaw, Lynn Meyer, Pat Pollock, and Mary Lee Settle. Special thanks to Dick Fredericks for wise and pointed advice, to Sam Vaughan for early counsel and encouragement, to Matthew Carnicelli for expert editing, and to Jane Gelfman for her patient, unflagging interest. Heartfelt thanks to my husband, George Garrett, for his life-sustaining humor and enthusiasm.

AUTHOR'S NOTE

This book is a narrative based on fact and memory, set in a small hospital during the 1980s. The characters are composites, with the exception of Paul Bengtson, Jud Knox, and Carolyn Roberts, who appear as themselves. In that decade I was privileged to hold a sequence of management positions in three hospitals of different size and purpose—two community hospitals and a university teaching hospital. My narrator, who tells this story, works in one, the smallest. I chose to keep her there, to give the issues a continuing base in one setting.

The admiration I hold for all who work in small hospitals and my personal regard for former colleagues in New England, especially in Maine, know no bounds.

Something will come to you.
RICHARD WILBUR, "Walking to Sleep"

I know what happens in my neighborhood
By sounds, by heart.
GEORGE GARRETT, "Postcard"

ONE

I am a tall woman with a quiet approach to management, inclined to observe a situation before taking action. To see the faces of the others seated at the table and to hear what they say, I sit with my back straight up, leaning forward. The chairs around the table are all armchairs, wide and comfortable and made of dark polished wood like silk to the touch, all touching arm to arm so that one person getting up and leaving causes much scraping and moving of chairs. Under the harsh ceiling light of the meeting room we appear more tired than we actually are and make allowances for this when we look at one another. The room is narrow, too narrow for this table and the dozen or so chairs crowded around it, too small for the shelves from floor to ceiling stacked with ten years of the *New England Journal of Medicine* and other medical and nursing journals. Two oil paintings cover the only wall space. They are quiet seascapes with rocks and sand in the foreground, painted by John Shipley, president of the board. Now they look almost worn by years of the half-attentive gaze of people in meetings. This room is also the medical library and the doctors' lunchroom. Most of the time a meeting of one kind or another is going on here.

Outside, the wind is high, the early dark held back by a lingering March sunset. A light snow covers the ground. Maine is cold in March, but here on the coast it is warmer than inland. The ocean warms the air.

I have been administrator of this seventy-nine-bed hospital for six years, and I could easily regret having come here in the first place, but I do not. It is a community general hospital, voluntary, not for profit, independent, governed by a local board of trustees. It takes in strangers as if they were its own. We run it like a business, competitive and flush with specialists, pushing the limits of its funds to buy the latest and best medical technology. A microcosm of American health care. But I am afraid for it. Financially we are breaking even, but for how long? All over the country small hospitals are closing. Last year forty-five hospitals closed, two of them in Maine.

We are in a meeting of the strategic planning committee. Its subject is the purpose, breadth, intensity, volume, cost, and means of hospital care. Regardless of the new language— "establish a mission, assess the environment, analyze strengths and weaknesses, examine constraints, decide on strategy, come up with specific objectives"—the meeting has been going on since the founding of the hospital eighty-some years ago, or so it seems.

My former colleagues in city hospitals told me, when I left them to come here, that I was making a mistake.

"You will disappear into a backwater. You'll be stuck."

"Perhaps."

"Are you running away?"

"Something like that."

"What you're doing, you know, is lying down on the sand and letting the tide wash you away."

As it turns out, I do not miss big city hospitals. They are fine places, do not misunderstand me. If you are ill and go into one, your chances are good. But there is an awkwardness to a place where a patient's name is written down over and over, spelled again and repeated once more because no one already knows it, and even after the patient has been in the hospital for several days, still no one knows it. Awkward and unwieldy, to let specialty departments draw lines around themselves like the old Berlin Wall, cross at your peril. If city hospitals have an underlying order, it comes from the turf battles themselves creating their own gravity and holding all parts to the center in centripetal rage. I told my colleagues I was leaving because I wanted my own shop. Every hospital manager wants his or her "own shop," knowing all the time that nothing in the management of a hospital is one's own and everything important is done by others. Still, we work under the illusion that if granted the privilege to take action, we could configure the ideal hospital. My colleagues said that when one is dreaming about making a difference in health care, it's better to be young. I was not young; I was fifty. I would regret leaving the center of health care, they said, and moving to the fringe.

At the head of the table Jack Mathias is saying it's up to the rich to take care of the poor; they've been doing that in their own way since the founding of the hospital near the turn of the century (by his grandfather, he always reminds us). Jack is a thin, angular man who could have been chipped out of the large granite freestanding rock near the front entrance of the 1958 building and given life with the covenant that he stay forever within a few hundred yards of his motherstone. And he has; he has obeyed: has stayed here in town all his life except for one interruption, the Second World War. Jack fought in the infantry from Casablanca across North Africa, up through Sicily, and onto the Italian mainland. He was wounded near Cassino and witnessed the bombing of the monastery there, which he will tell you about if you ask him, and once he has your attention he will take his story further, to the destruction of charitable hospitals by the very forces that were put in place to preserve them. For forty-three years he has sold insurance in a small office on the main street of town and served on the board of trustees of the hospital, twice as president, most often as treasurer. He is treasurer now. He would rather be treasurer than president.

Tony Phalen, former administrator of this hospital, now a trustee, interrupts Jack to note that here in Maine, and in general, there are more poor than rich, but then an innovative hospital can serve both. I admire Tony. He is a smiling, bright man of seventy with forty-six years of experience in this business—a mischievous man, at his best when playing games, although serious, always, about medical care. Tony came here fifteen years ago to retire, but the hospital needed help in those days, he told me, and the job looked like so much fun he couldn't resist. Picking up his lead has been a common temptation for me. Often I have thought I could learn to manage a hospital by watching Tony, imitating him like an art student copying stroke for stroke the paintings of an old master. And I believed myself smart enough to use only the best of his strokes and ignore the rest. But imitating Tony is impossible, I know that. We are opposites. I manage by consensus. Tony stirs things up. The best ideas come out of chaos, he says. He is ahead of his time.

"It's a matter of marketing," Tony is saying, "and by that I mean finding out what people want and how they want it and then finding a way to give it to them"—sometimes Tony throws a curveball—"at the same time choosing the most lucrative hospital services, as the for-profit chains do, take Humana, for instance, they know what it's about, risk and venture and a positive revenue flow, even a profit, well, for us, not exactly a profit, we are a not-for-profit hospital, but you know what I mean, a contribution to the future. Now, I have a heart condition, you see, and if there were a cardiologist at this hospital with the up-to-date technology that goes with the practice of heart specialists, then I could stay here in the familiar surroundings that enhance my health. Those who are growing old should have the latest technology right in their own community."

Next to Tony is Sidney James, M.D., general and vascular surgeon. A tall man in his forties with smooth, clear skin and no expression, blue eyes fastening onto you while at the same time looking through and beyond you to something else. On a snow-covered afternoon seven years ago Dr. James drove up to the door of the hospital, and it was Tony's luck that he was in his office with the door wide open at the moment Sidney James walked in. If Tony had been out, Dr. James would have gone on up the road because at that time in his life it did not matter to him exactly where he was. He left behind a medical center practice and a divorce, piled everything he owned into the back of his car, and drove from Southern California in a diagonal line from southwest to northeast across the country from one coast to another. Ours was the hospital nearest to the point where he could no longer follow that diagonal line without driving into the Atlantic Ocean. He and Tony recognized each other instantly: a couple of weathered pros who had come here for a reason, to use the hospital for their own purposes but not entirely, because the place, the hospital and the town together, needed them as much as they needed the place. In a few seconds these two men knew they could be enormously useful to each other. Dr. James got a license to practice in Maine (no trouble, he had an impeccable record), and the board granted him privileges to practice surgery in the hospital. He opened an office, bought a small house on the river, married a local woman, and took superb care of his patients.

"Never in a million years could we recruit a surgeon like James to a hospital like this!" Tony had said.

Dr. James is speaking carefully in a soft and patient voice, as if to a gathering of children, about the immediate need for certain items of surgical equipment. "It's a long list, and expensive, as you will see, and of course, if I *have* to operate without these, I will, but since you are considering a strategy for the future, I advise you not to ignore the potential of an active surgical service."

Too active. The events of the day are fresh in my mind. Such hell broke loose in the operating room this morning over two missing surgical instruments that the nurse supervisor, Linda LeMay, quit on the spot. Dr. James was well along in his first case, an abdominal aortic aneurysm repair, a complicated procedure, when he saw that his open set of sterile instruments lacked two important items. The circulating nurse, Fran Page, hurried out to find the instruments and run them through the autoclave and bring them to the operating table, where Dr. James stood by the open wound, carefully controlling his rage. He has extraordinary control. He finished the operation, closed the wound, and followed the patient to Recovery. When he returned to the operating room, he took the pale green sheets from the table and tore each one carefully in half, then in quarters, then in long, thin strips, which he draped with mock gentleness side by side over the anesthesia machine. Dr. Hart, a quiet man even for an anesthesiologist, said under his breath that if Dr. James put one more linen strip on his anesthesia machine, he would kill him. Fran gathered up the strips one by one while Dr. James draped several more over the operating lights mounted to the ceiling. Martha Bonnier, R.N., grabbed the strips from the lights before they caught on fire. Fran hurried out to the alcove to pull the plug from the scrub sink, where Dr. James had turned on both faucets to let the sink fill with water and overflow. Martha and Fran prepared the OR for the next patient, breaking their record for turnaround time. Dr. Cartwright, the new orthopedic surgeon, stood in the scrub alcove with his arms flung wide, singing in a fine baritone about sending in the clowns, then went to Linda's desk and tore the pages of the OR schedule notebook one by one into small pieces, explaining that his office schedule was now in pieces because of delay in starting this case, so why shouldn't the hospital's schedule be in pieces also? Linda cleaned out her desk and left.

". . . and a full-time technician assigned exclusively to my instruments." Dr. James speaks softly, so that the others at the table strain forward to listen. Now his tone is so matter-of-fact that his request becomes an obvious truth.

Could we lose this fine surgeon if we do not grant his request?

Tony says that quality in medical care resides in the skill of an individual physician. "What is there other than what a doctor does for his patient?"

Across the table is Bev Tracey, R.N., a young outdoorswoman, blond and capable, who will buttonhole you in the hall to tell you about a patient. She is telling us about Miss Jannsen.

". . . she is alone, you see, she has no family, sixty-six years old, no one comes to see her. Dr. Talley suspects a lung carcinoma, the X ray is negative, which could mean that the tumor is smaller than a half centimeter or else it is hiding, which means we have a chance if we act now, in the early stages, and he wants tests on her, a bronchoscopy, a CAT scan, a nuclear scan. The bronchoscopy we can do, but the mobile CAT scan truck is out for repairs, so to get these tests, you cannot *imagine* what it takes from here! We call the hospitals in Biddeford and Portland, in Portsmouth and Dover, New Hampshire, even Boston, and schedule her where we can, when the rescue squad can spare a driver for a whole day. Then we hone the trip down to a living inch: Biddeford is twenty-six point seven miles, Dover twenty-three and a quarter, Boston sixty-seven, Portland forty-four and a half. The road to Portland is wide but crowded, the roads to Dover narrow but not as long, you can drive to Boston on one straight road, but when you approach the city, it enters confusion, and time is lost, so we balance weather against distance, traffic against the urgency of the trip, the danger of speeding against bumps in the road, and who is driving. You see, every trip is a string of choices. Miss Janssen will wait three hours or more in the waiting room of one of the hospitals—some of them pay no attention to a patient from some little hospital over on the coast—then the tests, then the long trip back. Speaking of quality . . . Now, if we *belonged* to a big hospital, as part of its system and its revenue flow, as you say, then it would send a van for Miss Janssen because she is bread and butter for it, know what I mean?"

"And lose our independence?" Jack Mathias asks. "We know how to take care of our own here."

"Dr. Talley could send her to Portland overnight," Dr. James offers.

"She won't go. She clings to the bed rails with white knuckles as if she thinks we might force her, closes her eyes and wrenches her face into a frown, and makes little piping, squeaking sounds—'Peep peep peep!'—like that, until Dr. Talley lets her stay. She is afraid of strange places and especially of dying in a strange place. She is afraid of dying in her boarding home because she lives on the second floor and her body would have to be carried down the stairs slowly, with difficulty because of the narrow turn in the stairs—'They might drop me,' she says—past the dining room and parlor, where the other residents could peer out and see her, in a prostrate position, covered with a blanket but perhaps her feet not covered but extending from under the blanket, straight up, perhaps without shoes. It would be embarrassing, she says, to be seen by the other boarders who are not all that friendly even when one is alive. Do you get the picture?"

Coleman Forbes breaks the silence. "The picture is this: Consider the individual, at the same time the financial bottom line and the quality of medical care, as well as the needs of the community and a moral obligation to care for the uninsured. Nothing to it."

Coleman is a log of memory and a source for oral and written history, a modest man with bright eyes and a long face full of interest without flattery, energy without animation. After the Second World War he returned from the Navy, started a weekly newspaper here, *The Observer,* and published it for thirty-five years until he sold it one day on the spur of the moment to a young woman just graduated from New York University who wanted to begin her journalism career in a small town rooted in basic American values. Every day, except in heavy snow, Coleman rides his bicycle through the length of town, down Organug Road to Sewall's Bridge, through the woods to the shore road and along the stretch around the harbor, then back over the river bridge to the post office, to the bank, to Rick's (All Seasons) Restaurant for coffee. Wherever there is construction or an outdoor project—a new roof going onto the Harbor Inn, a barge dredging the harbor, a new sewer line, a new fire station—he stops and watches, leaning on the handlebars of his bicycle, exchanging stories with those who like to tell and hear them. Every afternoon he parks his bicycle against the white birch tree outside my office window and checks in to see if we are still in business. Often, at the end of the day, I ask Coleman how hospitals got into this fix.

"History is a stubborn shadow; it stays with hospitals; there is no escape," he says.

Then he tells me about one or another moment or event in the past that has dogged the hospital ever since. Almost always at the center of that moment is Dr. Josiah Cage, who at the turn of the century came to this town and convinced Jack's grandfather and other courageous town citizens to establish a hospital for the practice of scientific medicine, "according to rational methods and established fact." Coleman often brings me pages from the earliest records, carefully preserved. Here is Dr. Cage's response to his fellow founders when they asked him to define a hospital:

—where a physician practices scientific medicine by observation of the patient, the keeping of records, and instruction of nurses.

—for a patient without family; and for removal of a patient from a family who fail to follow instructions.

—to concentrate on the disease itself, rather than the circumstances of the patient.

—for convenience of nursing care under physician orders followed promptly; to guarantee rest and cleanliness, control diet and medicines.

—for travelers, when ill.

—where citizens with time to spare find useful tasks to occupy their day and enjoy a nobility of service without recompense.

—with a sterile place for surgery.

—not an almshouse.

"Cage used to say that science and the welfare of the patient walk hand in hand, like inseparable twins," Coleman tells me. "He admired the End Result Idea of Dr. Ernest Amory Codman, a surgeon who practiced at Massachusetts General Hospital around the year 1913. It was simply this: that a hospital should follow every patient it treats long enough to know the success of the treatment. 'If it was not successful, we should know why not,' he said. A simple matter."

Now at the meeting Coleman is saying that history shadows hospitals for a reason. There are ideas to be drawn from it, and the best strategy is to study the mistakes found in history and plan carefully around them.

Arthur Seiler, M.D., is laughing out loud. The lapels of his big plaid horse blanket of a jacket are bouncing with laughter. His jacket is the only color at the table, its red and blue and green squares and big brown leather buttons heightened by the pitiless overhead light. Art Seiler is a general practitioner, a short, heavy man, light on his feet, who in 1950 set up practice in a house on the main street of town when the only other doctor here was Josiah Cage, who was approaching his eightieth birthday. Patients left old Dr. Cage and flocked to the new young Dr. Seiler. In his glory days Art Seiler's practice took in at one time or another most of the four thousand people in town and some from the county whose population in total numbers was twice that if you consider the farther sections north and west. To have a successful practice (alone, solo, never with a partner), and to discourage younger doctors from coming here, he covered the emergency room, rode the ambulance, remembered the names of children, visited the old people in the suffocating patched-up back rooms off their children's kitchens, served as town health officer. Now he is losing a few patients to the young internists and family practitioners who have recently set up practices in town. Every morning he stops by the admitting office and runs his eyes down the handwritten list of patients admitted to the hospital, the name of the admitting doctor entered next to each name, checking to see who among his patients has left him for a new doctor. All meetings make Art Seiler laugh, and this one especially. The very notion that planning could affect the future . . .

"What good is planning? Can it prevent the unexpected? What good is a half-baked idea from the past? You might dream up things to improve the present, since we're stuck with it."

"What things?"

"If you have to ask, then you can't be told."

"Tell us."

"Well, if you are hit with a flu epidemic like the one in 1918—Cage told me about it; twenty-nine patients in the old hospital on cots in the halls and parlor, others at home waiting for someone in the hospital to die and free up a cot; he said he had never seen people so sick out of all proportion to their symptoms, and Cage couldn't handle it, the nurses couldn't handle it; they got fishermen to leave their boats and carry the bodies down the stairs and out to the funeral parlor, four trips a day, four funerals a day for three weeks—then you forget the past and the future and do what Cage did: arrange to have straw spread over the streets to muffle the sound of the hearse. You might turn your strategic planning to some gestures of this kind.

"Now, we have a serious problem. The path leading to the business cottage has no handrail, and my patients who walk up the path to the cottage to pay their bills are in danger of falling. I request immediate installation of a handrail."

It is late, the cafeteria next to the meeting room is quiet, and outside, the sky is dark. Through the window I can see the tall amber lights of the new parking lot and the entrance to the emergency room, where the high-beam headlights of the ambulance shine toward me. The attendants are bringing in a patient, but because of the light in my eyes, I cannot see who it is.

At this hour the group around the table should be restless and pushing back chairs to leave, but everyone stays, held together by a discussion, now lively, of whether the handrail should be made of wood or metal pipe, should it curve with the path? That would cost more than straightening the path itself and lining it on either side with a straight handrail.

Perhaps we will survive after all.

Two

Spring does not come to Maine. I have learned to forget about it; it is not a factor. But this morning there is enough of an ocean breeze to draw me out early and send me walking to work the long way, along the river. As I come out of the woods near Hancock Wharf, I see Tim Bailey walking toward town with his steady, unchanging gait, a short and careful stride as if each step were a life decision. Tim is a regular in the hospital. At Christmas and in bad weather, you can count on him. He comes to the emergency room every Christmas Eve short of breath with heavy chest pain. The doctor on duty admits him to the hospital, relieves his symptoms, and Tim has a bed and meals and friendly faces for Christmas. Tim's registration card shows a different address each time—"The Piney Wood Motel Annex" or "RR19, Box 4." There is no Rural Delivery Route 19 here. You can count on Tim in other seasons, too. In late summer and early fall I sometimes see him, in his dark green work shirt and trousers and a cap that says "Bama Feed" on the front, curled up asleep near the rocks at the north end of the beach under the secure shadow of a fine many-windowed mansion with solid stone foundation and an umbrella-decked terrace—the summer club of the summer colony. Tim is wiry with olive skin and a dark beard, and you can spot him on the road a long way off by the determined force of his step. He is old enough to have been in Vietnam. Almost always he walks the same route: north along the Long Sands beach to Short Sands and inland on the Cage Road (named not for Dr. Cage but for a man who kept a llama in a cage in front of his house near the edge of the road, years ago) to Route 1, then left on Mountain Road, climbing slowly toward Mount Agamenticus (not what you would call a real mountain, more like a hill in a flat landscape). As he climbs, he leaves behind the circumspect tight-box houses of white or dark red clapboard, dark gray or green shingles, that line the lower roads, and walks past poorer places—shacks and trailers with nine or more half-rusted cars parked in front, each one gutted for its parts, and abandoned trailers isolated on scrub land with stubble for grass. Where do the homeless sleep in this part of the world? Anywhere empty and silent. He passes the half-built frame of a box house set on mud soil exposed and waiting for new grass to take hold, then a stretch of woods, then one or two isolated houses painted bright turquoise or yellow. These could be in a suburb on a street with lawns and a sidewalk except that if you go inside, you will see one room and a dirt floor and maybe eight or ten people living there. When the blacktop turns toward the mountain summit, Tim leaves it for a dirt road through deep, quiet woods, several miles of woods not within sight of but near the site-to-be of a new industrial plant that will manufacture airplane parts and create six hundred new jobs (at least that is what we hear). Soon Tim sees the west bank of the reservoir, then woods again. Do you sleep on the edge of the curving reservoir, Tim? Do you miss the water when you are miles inland? Now coming to Mill Lane, crossing Cider Hill Road onto Birch Hill, past small farms of cornfields and hay and a few cows on land cleared from pine and maple woods, then onto Beech Ridge Road to South Side, the houses turning handsomer as Tim approaches the sea, over Sewall's Bridge and up Lindsay Road, where we are now, Tim walking ahead of me.

Did I say Tim always walks the same route? That is an extension of the truth. Sometimes he turns right, onto Cider Hill Road, to the landfill. Is this where he finds food? If Tim should walk in that direction for a long time, he would come to a shoe factory that makes a fine-quality leather shoe of the Oxford type with laces and a firm sole, sturdy and well constructed. A pair of shoes made in New England will last you a long time. Sometimes he turns left, following Cider Hill Road past more farmhouses, many connected to barns of their own by sheds that are both outer storage and passageway, cool in summer and protected in winter. Does anyone know you well enough, Tim, to invite you to sleep in one of those house-to-barn sheds? Tim has walked his routes enough to know where he can sleep.

Now we are approaching the center of town. Ahead of us are the old graveyard and, beyond that, the generous and perfectly proportioned white Congregational church, built large enough to hold everyone in town. We pass a cluster of eighteenth-century houses of dark red and mustard yellow clapboard, tight boxes with central chimneys. Two have additions of odd shapes, as if the original boxes were built to hold on to anyone's whim of design. One house is a museum. On my visits there I can feel the dark warmth and cell-like safety of rooms built by the early settlers against fear and cold on the edge of a strange land. Early history is alive here: the past and present live side by side in ordinary confusion. New Englanders are frugal; they use what they have, and the past is part of what they have. The early history of Maine is filled with accounts of danger, of whole communities (both Indians and settlers) tricked and slaughtered. In that hostile environment the people of Maine formed townships with a form of government that suited their situation. Town government requires a lot of participation from local citizens. Under the deafening roar of bullheaded argument at town meeting there is a local public spirit, an attachment, a feeling of power and independence close to home.

Tim is turning into the hospital driveway. Is it symptoms of a heart attack this morning, Tim? Are you truly ill this time? Or is a storm coming? The morning is beautiful, the weather fine. But it is April. April is tricky. There are two months to watch out for in Maine: April and November. In late April, after a long winter, when the ground offers nothing but mud, and in November, after the leaves have fallen and winter stretches too far ahead, people behave erratically, write long, urgent letters, give in to outbursts and make foolish decisions. Then, when Thanksgiving comes, and again when the June lilacs bloom, reason returns. On the surface here time moves slowly with no sense of urgency.

Tim walks to the emergency room entrance, and I go in a different direction. Later I will inquire about him. Gerry Lebeau, director of nursing, is waiting outside my office. Gerry is a handsome woman, tired and single-minded, most of the time either passively hostile or simply reserving judgment. She will want to go above and beyond her budget to recruit a replacement for Linda LeMay, the operating room supervisor who quit on the spot. Gerry often stays at work later than I do and often comes in earlier in the morning, as if she thinks we are in a contest over who can show the most selfless devotion to the hospital. Right now she sits on top of our secretary's desk with her coffee mug and a sheaf of papers, looking as if she has been there for several long hours made uncomfortable by my failure to arrive and open my office.

"I have an applicant for the position of operating room supervisor, a nurse from Florida. She is qualified; she will keep order. She wants thirty-nine thousand."

"Too much. Can you promote from within?"

"No one here is material for management."

"Redefine material."

"You would sacrifice quality to stay within a budget?"

"Quality appears to be for sale."

We sit in silence. Bone shadows circle her eyes; lines of fatigue cover her flat, hard face. A fast reel of the long years she has worked in this hospital plays over it. Long years full of daily decisions. She is the one who has balanced cost and quality in this place, not I. I want to make her working life easier. She needs that nurse from Florida, someone with a fresh point of view, fresh air from the South. The operating room is a vulnerable flank where serious mistakes can happen. The first part of quality is order.

"Does the Florida nurse want to come here?"

Gerry's expression changes very slightly, but I can see the change. The lines in her face soften; there is the barest shadow of a smile, enough relaxing of muscles and beginning of eyes glazing over, the barest hint of boredom and a trace of disappointment tagged onto her obvious relief that the operating room might become manageable after all. She thinks she has won but too easily, without a fight. I am a pushover.

"Of course, if you hire her you will have to cut at least a position and a half somewhere else . . ."

The cost of hospital care has been rising by 8 percent a year, faster than other parts of the economy. The consumer price index itself stays close to a yearly 3 percent increase.

Where do we cut our cost? Much of it is in salaries, wages, benefits. What should we do? Reduce staff to the minimum? People here expect their hospital to stand by, ready at all times to handle the unexpected. Send nurses home without pay when the hospital census falls? Then find them cheerfully ready to return to work when the census rises? A risk. We do not welcome risk.

Gerry leaves the room. Quick, while she is gone, here is another idea. Cross-train all the specialists, so that a nurse schooled in cardiac care also knows obstetrics, pharmacists move with ease into the clinical lab to cover the blood bank, a respiratory therapist dispenses medicines and works the emergency room, operating room nurses rotate three weeks on the long-term care unit. Change the incentives for the burrowing mammals who dig tunnel walls around their thin bodies of knowledge and look inward for status from their own professional groups in imitation of medicine, now so specialized it is losing sight of the territory. Change the source of status, so that the broader your training, the more recognition you receive. This could save millions of dollars in the nation's hospitals. But it is impractical and a risk. The way the hospital is configured now, quality is equal to deep and narrow specialty. A person taking care of a patient must have all the training, degrees, certifications, licenses, qualifications, and experience that protect the public from incompetence. Someone trained in two specialties might come up short of some knowledge or skill in one—causing an error. One serious error can harm a patient and close the hospital. Could we weather a malpractice suit? Everyone within twenty-five miles on three sides of us would know every detail of a malpractice suit within a matter of hours. Our reputation is good but fragile. The cost of defense lawyers would rise like a slag heap in front of the door and bury us.

Take the evening last week. Charlene Davis, R.N., was staffing the emergency room alone. No one could be spared from the floors to help her. Jim Boze came on at 3:00 P.M. to work until 11:00, the busiest hours. Jim Boze is a local boy trained as an emergency medical technician. An EMT can substitute for a nurse if no nurse is at hand, but better than that, Jim is good. He is good on the rescue squad, doesn't panic, can cut through the metal of an overturned car with one clean sweep of the saw and bring out the passengers one by one in correct position with every limb lined up as it should be, head stable, the body level, not hurrying but not wasting a single stroke or movement, like a first-class surgeon. It's remarkable that he is so good at ambulance work, being new at it. Fast on his feet and bright, and he'll do what Charlene tells him. We are likely to trust someone that good. But now and then Jim becomes pretty cocksure that he knows a lot about medicine and nursing care and makes a judgment on his own, in an understandable and quite natural response to the frontier atmosphere of this emergency room. Like being on the front line. Late in the evening a young couple traveling from Minnesota came in with their three-month-old baby. Dr. Anderson examined the baby and ordered a shot of Vistaril. Charlene had been called upstairs, so Jim went ahead and gave the baby a shot—the parents were impatient, you see, and did not like waiting—but he pulled the wrong vial, gave the wrong medicine. It was Valium instead of Vistaril. The parents took the baby back to their motel room, and two hours later Jim discovered his mistake and called them, telling them to bring the baby back in, a mistake had been made. He called Dr. Anderson, and Dr. Anderson called Dr. Witter, a pediatrician who lives forty miles away, and asked him to come in and take care of the baby, and he did, and the baby was fine, just slept longer than usual but was fine. We kept him here an extra day for observation, and the parents came and stayed in the room with him. All was well, you see. But the parents were wild with fear. They came to my office that first morning and talked for a long time to relieve the terror of the mistake, and I understood that and listened as they talked about Jim Boze. Why was he allowed in the emergency room if he was capable of an error like that? Did we always have such people in the emergency room? How about the rest of the hospital? What kind of hospital is this? Yes, it was good he saw his mistake and called them right away, but suppose he hadn't? Did you know when you hired him that he would call, that he has a record of calling about his own mistakes? Suppose you had hired someone who *wouldn't* have called. Then what? Suppose you have other employees who wouldn't have called. Have you screened everyone in your hospital? How about your weekend staff? How well do you know every single person who works here? Can you trust everyone to call in his or her mistake? What are you prepared to do about this, to make up for the anguish we have been through? *Cancel the bill?* Is that all you can think of to do for us? What kind of place *is* this? A lot of that time they stared at me without talking. When they came back at eight o'clock the next morning, I canceled all appointments and sat with them through the day, and when the third morning came and they turned up again, I was tempted to tell them I had given them all the time I could, but I did not, because I felt their pain and I feared a suit against the hospital—for negligence, for improper staffing, for lack of supervision of persons administering medication, for causing pain and anguish. They sat quietly in my office, saying that the baby was fine, that they were leaving and hoped never to come back here again as long as they lived, hoped I would improve the care in my hospital, so that others would never have the same terrible experience they'd had to endure. Then they were gone.

The fact that they are gone does not mean they will not sue. It means they left with a good result and no bill to pay.

There are plenty of reasons for not reconfiguring the health care system. It is a risk. We are too busy. We might make a mistake. People would have to stop being sick to let us get started.

* * *

Pete Roberge, director of finance, comes in carrying stacks of green spreadsheets that cover him up. A compact, ambitious young man, Pete would like to move on from this hospital to bigger and better things, leaving a strong shop behind him, for the record.

"The four percent margin we budgeted for the year is gone, zip, out of here." Pete half believes this is his fault. If he had more information, more minutely detailed cost data (he will cost out Miss Jannsen's trip to Portland, if she goes, down to the last tire scrape), then he could (he thinks) analyze us into financial health. We have spent all remaining endowment income for the year (Jack as treasurer keeps the larger portion to pay for charity care for some of our own worthy poor, as he describes the uninsured) on a new computer with the latest financial software. Now the computer is down, so Pete crunches numbers at home at night with a hand calculator, hours of work every evening, which is, after all, his children's time, his family comes first, but as he says, if we don't have the numbers, the hospital will go belly-up. Numbers pound in his head like heavy metal. The numbers are not good. We are running half full, half empty.

". . . Medicare patients, seventy percent of admissions . . ." Pete is saying.

The town is growing older.

We blame Medicare, instead of ourselves, for the trouble we're having. Medicare is the federal insurance program for all persons age sixty-five or older. From 1966 to 1983 Medicare paid hospitals "reasonable" costs for care of Medicare beneficiaries *after* the costs had been incurred. It was an open faucet. During that eighteen-year period hospital costs rose from $13.9 billion to $150 billion, an increase of 979 percent. (For the same period the consumer price index rose 242 percent.)

Now Medicare pays hospitals a predetermined fee per case, based on the patient's diagnosis and the group to which the diagnosis is related. There are 477 diagnosis-related groups. For Miss Jannsen, who may have lung cancer (DRG 82), Medicare will pay $4,032, an amount predetermined according to "standard" tests and treatment, hours of staff time, and average number of days in the hospital for a typical patient of that category.

The idea behind prospective payment, the *incentive,* is that hospitals will treat patients with close attention, speed, and efficiency, with costs lower than the amount of the fixed Medicare payment. Those that achieve good results through cost-conscious care will become stronger, able to compete for patients. Those that cannot will close.

But prospective payment and the pigeonholing of patients into categories create conflicting incentives. There is the incentive to skim, or to provide hospital care that is so efficient it could be less than the patient needs—that is, discharge Miss Jannsen from the hospital when she is *almost* ready, bring the cost of her case in under the amount of the payment, and retain the difference. Then there is the opposite incentive: to do more for a patient than may be necessary on the chance that certain tests will reveal a condition that takes the patient into a "higher" diagnostic group, bringing with it a higher fee per case.

For Pete and for me, the temptation (incentive) is to get right down into the middle of medicine and influence how many days the patient can stay, what kinds of X rays, how many lab tests. Always in the past medicine has made the decisions and hospitals have followed them. But now, with the key to cost control lying somewhere deep within medical practice, it is not farfetched to imagine Pete sitting down with Dr. Sidney James over coffee and making suggestions about his use of instruments, the time he takes with a particular case in the operating room, or his diagnosis and the ramifications of it in the DRG hierarchy. Dr. James would leave, of course—pack up his car and his family and drive off in some diagonal direction, a sharp-angled line to a large hospital in the Southwest, perhaps, but he would find the same thing there, though handled in a more discreet and sophisticated manner. (According to Art Seiler, Pete and I are bumpkins. If we were really good at managing a hospital, we wouldn't be *here,* he tells us, adding that the key to cost control lies not in medicine but deep within administration.) Anywhere Dr. James goes he will find the same pressure on doctors to "maximize reimbursement" to the hospital, the same over-the-shoulder scrutiny of doctors' mode of practice. He might as well stay with us.

Prospective payment was designed by academics to change hospital behavior. It fails because of the presence of conflicting incentives—to do too little, to do too much—and because it is blind to the nature of medical practice, the uncertainty that follows physicians like a demon. Not absolutely sure of what they are looking for, fearful that their diagnostic route will take a wrong turn, and, most of all, deeply desirous of a good result, physicians are weighed down by uncertainty, and beyond that, they believe that if outsiders are permitted to see this, medicine will lose its political power. (It will, but not for that reason.) Physicians see nonphysicians as limited in intellect. They assume that we cannot comprehend the whole; that we look at weakness, not at strength; that we are ungrateful. Not so. The opposite is true. We respect, admire, appreciate.

Hospitals respond to incentives, insulting as they are, like anyone else caught between trying to do the best for patients and running a business. What would mitigate, for us, the sense that we act only in our own self-interest, and only for short-term revenue gain, is the thought that by a tooth-and-nail fight to be efficient in a maze of uncertainty we would make a contribution to the future, make some difference to the long-term health of the people here, even shrink the system enough to cover the uninsured.

". . . change the mix . . ." Pete is saying.

Does he mean the "mix" of rich and poor, old and young, insured and uninsured? Coleman tells a story about Dr. Cage, who in 1905 persuaded the other founders that a hospital is not an almshouse. " 'We will care for the rich and the poor at the same time,' Cage said. 'I charge no fee to the poor as they often have interesting diseases to contribute to the advancement of scientific medicine. The rich, without being aware of it, will pay enough to cover the expenses of the poor, leaving a small profit for the hospital.' Jack Mathias's grandfather stood at the top of the stairs and shouted that this was the last straw; he could not stand idly by and watch the hospital make a profit over the diseased bodies of his neighbors. Cage assured him it was not exactly a profit but a contribution to the future."

"... shift the costs ..." Pete says. From the poor to the rich? We have played the cost-shifting game, piling the costs not paid by Medicare and Medicaid and Blue Cross onto the backs of self-insured paying patients.

"... change the *case* mix ..." Pete says.

With layers of cost data buried in the computer Pete can analyze "product lines," such as lung cancer, to learn which cases will cost us less than what Medicare will pay. If one of our own is ill with an unprofitable illness, does the hospital urge the doctor to admit him or her elsewhere? The incentive is there. On the other hand, if Pete finds a profitable product line, we are inclined to recruit a physician who will admit many patients with that diagnosis.

In a vortex of conflicting incentives like these, the likely thing to do is to steer straight ahead with an eye on the individual patient.

"... or invite a large hospital to take us over," Pete offers.

This would be difficult. Even if we were strong—a desirable acquisition—Jack Mathias would offer his dead body stretched across the meeting room table. According to Coleman, there has been talk of mergers in the past, and each time Jack scraped back his armchair and threw his arms and chest forward onto the table and remained silent with his head down until the others agreed to reject the idea.

"So we'll serve the elderly. With a cardiologist—"

Pete groans. "I've costed it out. We can't afford the equipment: first a Holter monitor, then an echocardiography machine, and then he or she will want to do cardiac catheterization—you watch, we're in for a *cascade* of capital investment."

According to Tony, we should think about quality, not cost. "Quality brings volume; volume brings revenue; revenue covers cost," he likes to say. When volume is low, economies of scale are lost, and beyond that, the skill of the individual physician is at stake. A surgeon like Sidney James must keep his hand in. So must a cardiologist. The more cases a doctor has, the more likely his skills are well honed. But (and here is

Tony's point) we can defy the laws of volume by recruiting the best cardiologist and "marketing" him or her in order to attract a large number of patients, so that the presence of quality becomes the reason for the volume, not the other way around. Should we hustle health care like a commodity?

Pete and I talk about Miss Jannsen, who will stay longer than the eleven days figured into DRG 82, who does not want to go to Augusta for a scan, and who, if she stays here a long time, will cause us to lose money. I tell Pete it is a serious quality issue, to urge Dr. Talley to discharge Miss Jannsen too soon, and he agrees but points out that this aspect of quality leads to the closing of the hospital.

We exchange statements of consolation.

"Our birthing rooms are the largest in the state, big enough for a husband and friends and maybe the whole town to be present at the birth."

"The alcohol counseling program has really taken off. There are more alcoholics in town than we had any idea, some who can pay."

"Everyone says the new internist, Dr. Anderson, is first-rate."

And best of all: "Summer is coming." In summer the town is filled with tourists. And the summer residents arrive for the season, from Boston and Providence and Philadelphia, and open their "cottages"—those mansions of white or brown shingles or yellow stucco, each with a flagpole and a host of pink geraniums, set high on the edge of the cliff overlooking the ocean. We know summer is here when dark green canvas awnings spring suddenly from the windows of the cottages and American flags rise to hold their own in the ocean breeze. Every year Jack Mathias watches for the arrival of the summer people and hardly lets them unpack their tennis rackets before he is calling on them to ask for money for the hospital. From his careful study of the daily lists of admissions he knows who has come to this hospital, and from conversations with Gerry he knows who has fared well and who has not. The rich should take care of the poor, he reminds us.

Pete and I look forward to summer, when for three months the hospital is filled to the brim. Then, when the leaves fall, the census falls, too. Not that we want people to fall ill, do not misunderstand. It is simply that we have let incentives set by others put us on the course we are on, and if you are going to have to be cared for in a hospital, we hope you will come to us.

Always at lunch there is a crowd of doctors in the meeting room and the talk is casual, mostly about wood stoves and wood, about boats and what needs fixing. Everyone's boat has something wrong with it at any given moment. Through their easy talk these doctors take collegial measure of one another, although an outsider like me would not know that without dropping in here often and hanging around for a while, at the risk of intruding. Dr. Talley, a pale, bald man with bright dark eyes who has kept traces of his Brooklyn accent, is hanging the wall phone receiver between his ear and shoulder while rocking his head from side to side with a silly grin and a Soupy Sales gesture of thumb to temple and fingers waving in the air, signaling me to stall the operator relentlessly paging him on the central loudspeaker. When he is not on the phone, he tells stories about his former patients in Brooklyn. "So I said, 'Mrs. Gotoff, you have liver cancer, and I am concerned about your hypertension and diabetes,' and she said, 'Well, as long as I have my health, I guess I'm okay. Right, Doctor?' " Dr. James joins the conversation when it turns to mountain climbing or canoeing on the Allagash River, which flows north, he always reminds us.

When the talk is about medicine and someone brings up a patient, the air shifts slightly, and in the shoptalk they seek and deliver information, some putting their own knowledge on display for several colleagues at once and others listening, evaluating, a way of learning without having to request a formal consult. The meeting room is a referral pit, the small hospital equivalent of the commodities exchange except that the actual referrals aren't made here—only the preliminary sizing up. From general and family practitioner to surgeon, from internist to surgeon, to obstetrician/gynecologist, to ear/nose/throat, always in the direction of specialty, rarely back to general or family practice, patients are referred first according to doctors' friendships, but those friendships are founded in the first place on professional trust, referred on the basis of the results of earlier referrals, then withheld on old or new resentments clothed in the language of judgment. Now and then a clique forms and boycotts a colleague. For instance, Drs. Talley and Burt have decided that Dr. James's perceived high-handedness is going to cost him, and they now refer all their patients to the new surgeon, Dr. Wing, who is agreeable and untested. A risk hidden in the happy glow of helping a new young colleague build his practice. Dr. Seiler, on the other hand, calls Dr. Wing an "Ivy" and refers his patients only to Dr. James, who has bailed him out of a couple of tight spots recently and whose arrogance he knows to be sadness in disguise.

I am not a physician and therefore cannot pretend to understand physician referral patterns, even though the future of the hospital depends on them.

If Dr. James loses referrals, he will leave. But I cannot interfere. Doctors are independent practitioners, members of a profession organized for self-government. The hospital gives them "privileges" to practice here, not employment. Bureaucratic lines of authority surround them but do not reach them in the usual way of organizations.

Also, these doctors are loners. They came here for the quiet and the professional freedom. And to escape something. Refugees, every one of them. Maine is full of refugees. The mystique of Maine has made it a haven for those in flight—from financial failure, divorce, other falls and setbacks—and for those who need a second chance. Some refugees try hard to feel at home in Maine by imitating too scrupulously what they believe are the traits and virtues of Maine natives, by being too independent, too frugal, driving too hard a bargain. These doctors will not talk openly to me about medicine. Nor do I expect them to. I take into account their normally closed professional world and then factor in the condition of the refugee: an inclination to protect what one has left. That they build walls around their extensive knowledge of medicine, and also around their uncertainty, is in no way surprising. They will not let me in, and why should they? They are here to get away from carping administrators and other grievous annoyances. In their minds the hospital is a doctors' workshop, only that, a convenient center where doctors can diagnose, order treatment, follow a patient's progress, and write observations in the record. Clearly without doctors there can be no hospital, and without good doctors here people will travel all the way to Sanford or Biddeford or even Boston for their medical care because most people can get a ride when they want it, and once doctors are perceived to be no good people will leave them in droves and the hospital will close. On the other hand, when good doctors hold us hostage—"Buy this new technology or I will leave you"—the hospital is caught like a fly in a web.

I have to find out what they need for the kind of medical practice that is not wasteful, that reduces uncertainty and leads to good results. A balance of cost and quality. That is why I hang around their table at lunchtime and often in the late afternoon, at the risk of intruding. I am hoping to learn something. Is there a way to eliminate waste in medicine? Do away with procedures that have no effect on the end result?

They might let down their guard for a moment to say what they think. And I will do the same and tell them again about the variations we find among their charts in the treatment of patients with similar conditions, variations also in outcomes. I will tell them that finding the "one best way" in medical treatment is a popular idea right now among health care experts who are busy writing "practice guidelines" for treatment of certain illnesses, other things about the patients being equal. Experts place efficiency at the heart of quality. Scientific management has caught up with medicine. Today Coleman has come by for lunch and sits down with me and the usual group—Art Seiler and Sidney James and Dr. Talley, Dr. Cartwright, the new orthopedic surgeon, Dr. Somerville, the pathologist, a few others. Coleman is in a talking mood, and in the silence that follows his boldness in sitting down at the doctors' table he tells a story:

"You see, my aunt was housekeeper in the old hospital, and when I was a small boy, she often asked me to clean the surgery room, and I would quickly find something else to do because I did not want to go in there. 'You need to know about it now, so you will not be surprised later,' she said. And I remember scrubbing the floor carefully, moving my scrub brush in circles in the way the trustee Jonathan Culbertson instructed me, according to principles of scientific management—to increase efficiency and ensure our survival. 'Time and motion studies,' he explained, 'can break down a task and determine the "one best way." For industry it increases profits, why shouldn't it do the same for us?' That's what he would say. I grasped the brush and began in the corner, scrubbing in circular motion diagonally across the floor in a series of small circles widening into larger ones. That way I could finish the floor with only a half bucket of water and a dab of soap and in five minutes instead of twenty. The floor was made of a porous tile, white squares and small clay-red diamond shapes, and I rubbed it with a cloth to make it shine, but it would not. I waxed and rubbed it over and over, but it would not shine. Then I turned to the mahogany instrument cabinet that filled the back wall from floor to ceiling and polished the already gleaming wood as vigorously as I could. . . ."

Eyes glaze over, but Coleman does not mind. He knows doctors well and knows that none of them is hearing a connection between his story and medical practice, or if they are, they dismiss it as lay talk. They are tired of so many things, among them the sound of my voice asking them to treat their patients efficiently and discharge them quickly. Am I a physician? they ask. Do I have intimate knowledge of each individual patient's medical condition? Have I ever been *sued*? Do I know what that *means*? Tired of hearing me say that we are joined together—hospital and physicians—and what affects one affects the other. That their choice of tests and procedures is at the heart of runaway health care costs. That they have my full cooperation in avoiding unnecessary care and assuring quality. Once I asked them if a hospital has to keep on buying the latest high-cost technology in order to achieve the best medical results. Dr. James stifled a yawn and rolled his eyes heavenward, and Dr. Talley laughed himself into a fit—I mean, bouncing off the wall—and said I needn't worry, the candy man would tell me what to do.

For me it's a matter of having to ask without being told. And ironically, it is the same for them. Day after day they confront their patients' conditions and ask in their minds for the truth, finding some answers but not all of them. Uncertainty stalks them like a relentless shadow; they are no more free of it than I am. Less free of it than anyone. How do I tell them that I know this? Would it make any difference?

So, they are thinking, if the administrator doesn't like the way I practice medicine, I will leave . . . except that now practice locations like this one (the ocean, the river, the quiet) are not so plentiful, not so easy to find. There are now too many doctors in the nation, with more coming out of medical schools every year. Perhaps they are fortunate to be on the staff of this hospital. Perhaps we have a card to play.

The loudspeaker relentlessly pages one doctor after another, and the wall phone rings with calls from patients at home—the "regulars" mostly, who have cleverly caught on to the routine enough to know what time their own doctors are likely to come in for lunch and who know by heart the extension number of the phone next to the doctors' table, so that without having to rely on the switchboard, they can call them directly. I am drawn in momentarily by the comfort of it. Survival seems possible. After all, people are ringing up on the telephone asking for help; the doors are open, the lights on. I play host, briefly, to a whole range of seductive feelings of safety and importance. This community needs its hospital. Wants it. Doesn't want to lose it. Would be hard-pressed to ask its people to drive the curving roads to Dover or the relentless turnpike to Portland or Augusta to other hospitals and then find themselves having to stay in one of them overnight, away from home. Will go to extremes to keep it open.

Three

Elizabeth Littlejohn comes into the meeting room, knowing she will find Dr. Seiler here at lunch. He leaves the table and, with an arm across her shoulder, steers her to the emergency room. She is nineteen, suffering from bulimia, and given to binges of eating followed by purges, over and over. When she appears in the emergency room, the doctor on duty admits her to the hospital for two or three nights, to keep her from dehydration and put her on a good diet, but after she leaves, it doesn't last. She is back the next week in the same wasted state. She has no insurance and pays nothing on her bill, which is now $76,000, nor does she qualify for Medicaid because somehow she has money, an income, which puts her above the poverty line. A bright girl, talkative when she has been here a day and feels better. Then she is gone, then back again. When I ask Dr. Seiler about her, he is elusive.

"Ha, you don't want to know, enjoy your ignorance."

"Tell me."

"Find out for yourself, you're so clever at sleuthing around."

The hospital admits her because there is nowhere else for her to go, but we seem to do her no good. The bill rises higher. She agrees to a payment plan, ten dollars a month, then at the end of the month there is no payment, so Maggie Healy in the business office calls her on the telephone. Sometimes her grandfather answers and says Elizabeth is not home, she is in the hospital, sick, why doesn't Maggie know that, doesn't she work there? Sometimes no one answers. Or the phone has been disconnected.

"Can you send her to Portland for a work-up?"

"No insurance. If you get her on Medicaid, they say, we'll take her. So far no luck."

"Our system is designed for acute care and surgery and emergencies, all wrong for chronic illness. Chronic patients fall through the *cracks*! You know this is true, Dr. Seiler, and you are the ideal choice to head up a chronic illness clinic in the hospital. Could you give a day a week to it on salary?"

"You don't understand. I have an office. Did you know that? Patients come to my office. Perhaps you didn't know that. It is the way I make my living. Now you know."

"Then you'll see Elizabeth in your office instead of sending her to the emergency room, where we absorb the unpaid bill?"

Dr. Seiler is angry and will remain so for a couple of weeks.

Elizabeth feels at home in the hospital because at all times there are anywhere from two to five members of the Littlejohn family here. Kevin Littlejohn is dying of AIDS in room 6, the private room overlooking the river, and Dr. Seiler wants Kevin to remain in that particular room even though it is specifically endowed by Mrs. Butterworth of the summer colony, who requests that it be reserved for her each season from June to September in case she needs it and who will be displeased when she finds out the room is occupied by an AIDS patient. Dr. Seiler says he referred Kevin to home care, but for home care to work, a patient first has to have a home. A dirt-floor shack with nine people living in one room won't cut it, he says. Kevin's cousin Tommy Littlejohn is also an inpatient. Tommy lost his right arm below the elbow and his right leg below the knee in a motorcycle accident when a double trailer truck swerved and forced him in front of a car that ran over him. Dr. Seiler has tried to transfer him to Boston, where he can have first-class rehabilitation, but he refuses to go on the grounds that he doesn't know anyone there. "How will I live among strangers without an arm and a leg?" he cries. Dr. Seiler tells

Tommy he is a good-looking kid and no one looks at arms and legs anyway, only at faces. "Strangers look at what is *missing!*" Tommy shouts. With his good arm he grabs hold of Bev and the other nurses and tries to pull them down onto the bed with him. His good arm is strong. One time John Ferry, plant maintenance engineer, and two of his assistants came in to free Bev from Tommy's stranglehold. Tommy shouts obscenities when he doesn't get his way. Once Jack Mathias was in the hall and heard his language. Jack came immediately to my office to report that Tommy needs to be sent to a mental hospital. No one in his right mind uses words like that. So far Dr. Seiler has not been able to persuade Tommy to go to Boston.

In the cafeteria Elizabeth's aunt Flora Littlejohn presides like a self-appointed cruise director as the only person keeping order in this chaos. This evening she directs me to a table near the window. Outside, an April storm (when did it begin?) has rain falling in sheets and a high wind blowing waves like low surf over the pools of water covering most of the parking lot. Inside, it is darker than usual. The walls are bare except for the outlines of a mural, a sylvan scene in one color and one dimension. The orange vinyl-covered chairs we ordered to enhance employee morale actually do add cheer to the cafeteria. Flora Littlejohn's white hair flies in every direction; the clasps of her torn galoshes rattle against one another; the hem of her old army overcoat is caught in one of them. Every day at lunch, and again at supper, she takes her place next to the pink-smocked volunteer at the cash register and directs everyone to a table as if she were the maître d'. Almost everyone dutifully sits at the table selected by Flora. The cafeteria is her social program as the town has no formal day program for the mentally disabled.

The Littlejohns belong to this community and are therefore factors in the life of the hospital, as are all the others—those who live nearby, some in families and others alone, some in circumstances worse than the Littlejohn family but less noticeable, a good many better off, making a living on lobster and fishing boats, small farms, small businesses, shops and tourist enterprises, real estate and construction. Many are old with incomes that let them live quietly, out of sight most of the time.

Some earn their money during the summer, cleaning and cooking and walking dogs and watering the geraniums of the summer cottages. Others are moderately well-off and join the board of the hospital. At the extreme is the summer colony itself, which arrives with the lilacs in June and covers the town for a few short weeks with smiling, bronzed, well-clad oh-so-healthy people, who, while they are here, allow us to see them walk to the post office, sail in the harbor, run like wildfire on the tennis court, such a sight of health and good living it almost burns our eyes, not being used to it.

"Don't be fooled by the sight of them," Tony says. "All that rich food all their lives, and different *kinds* of stress, you know, they need a cardiologist as much as the rest of us, certainly as much as the poor who live on a diet of fried potatoes and junk food, equally devastating." When Tony gets hold of an idea, he carries it forward.

But I am thinking mostly of those who live here the year round, individuals and families who form a community. Here is Carrie Williams, who has been called "a pillar," who is at this moment carrying a supper tray wobbling in her hands. It is too heavy for her. I wish Flora would slow down. Why does Flora have to lead Carrie to the most distant corner table? For the last year Carrie has come every evening to the hospital's two-dollar dinner for senior citizens. She is eighty-five, a spinster who lives alone on a farm where her father and grandfather lived before her. She stands straight and determined. Her features are sharp, friendly, critical.

Those who remember will tell you that Carrie was a pillar of the Church Committee for the Sprucing Up of the Graveyard on the Green, the Committee for Thanksgiving Baskets to the Poor, the Library Committee for Culture and Consciousness. She crocheted afghans for the patients in the Shipley Wing, visited shut-ins (bringing small animals to perch in their laps), founded the local branch of the Society for the Preservation of New England Antiquities, and led the fight to preserve the beach between the harbor and the rocks as a public park: *Everyone* needs access to the ocean, she said, locking horns with the summer people and their real estate interests, no small feat. And every summer she gathered a host of willing women to present a country fair on the green, a joyous celebration at the height of the season. The ladies wore colonial dresses, and some of the men wore broad hats and locked their arms and legs in mock punishment in the stocks in the front of the Old Gaol, to the laughter and shouts of bands of children, even some from the summer colony. And there were balloons and a country band, long tables with white tablecloths, where the ladies served lobster and steamed clams and corn on the cob on blue oval pottery plates, each with its own small round bowl of melted butter, and on other tables near the church steps there were apple, cherry, and lemon pies, cookies and cakes of all kinds, and a whole table of homemade candy. Carrie organized a special pet show for the children with a blue-ribbon prize for the most "appealing pet to show a distinctive personality." One year it went to Art Seiler's little boy for a small and unusual red-eyed armadillo, an animal not native to Maine ("brought here from away, from the Southwest," Coleman told me), even so showing a certain courage and tenacity that appealed to the judges. Art Seiler and Coleman Forbes always went to the fair and stayed quite a long time, enjoying themselves.

When I first came to town, Carrie called on me at home and right away took herself on a tour of our house. She was quick; she saw everything on the walls, in the bookshelves. The small silver pitcher in the dining room, would I sell it to her? I said it was not for sale. She said she hoped I knew how to run the hospital in a businesslike way. A week later she invited me to her house, and I drove west along Route 91 into a deep pink winter sunset behind stands of blue spruce and white birch lining the narrow road, to a white clapboard farmhouse with a dilapidated half barn behind it, in the driveway an impeccable black 1948 Chevrolet. I bent my head to enter the doorway. The low ceiling and small windows were like those of the eighteenth-century houses on the green, but something was different here. Would I like to look around? As we moved slowly through the house, I saw that the walls, every inch, were lined with cabinets. There were three corner cupboards and more wooden cabinets behind the sofa. One by one Carrie opened the cabinet doors, where inside were stacks of china—plates standing at the back of the shelves, plates stacked with teacups and bowls on top, teapots and pitchers and creamers, platters and covered dishes of Meissen and Lowestoft and blue and white Chinese export, English china with blue and gold borders, French china with gold initials. A sudden shaft of late afternoon sunlight through the window shone on a tall, delicately flowered Dresden coffeepot and several dozen small cups and saucers. Carrie watched me carefully. I said these were beautiful things; was it a family collection? I had never seen anything like it. In the dining room were silver pitchers and candlesticks, English and American, some very early, and one cupboard filled with American pewter bowls and plates and pitchers. More in the kitchen—crystal goblets, dozens of them. Does she love these things? I wondered. She looked at me, not at the objects, as she opened cabinet doors one at a time. And then suddenly I knew that everything in the house, although she never said so, was for sale, and that it wasn't only money she wanted, it was *commerce*—the act of buying, selling, trading, of negotiating and arguing and coming to terms, the business of the market. She longed for commerce and couldn't arrange it for herself, too proud to be a shopkeeper, not knowledgeable enough to be a dealer. I saw later that I could have offered to trade my pitcher for something of hers and she would have come alive and kept me there for hours, discussing its value and what choices I had, what would be a fair trade. There would be several possibilities, of course—one for one or perhaps a combination. If I had provided a market for her, just for an hour or two, I would have made a friend. But I didn't think of it at the time.

Now she seems frail, almost apprehensive. She may even be glad for Flora's large solid army-coated back forging a path through the crowd in the cafeteria. People say that Carrie has a social security check for a living, and the house and car, and the china collection.

This is a community hospital, we say. What will we do for Carrie? Will the community take care of its own? What is a community? The word is overused and seldom defined. We know that finding out what the *community* needs and wants from its hospital, keeping eyes and ears open, leads to survival and success. But a definition? Most people believe they already know what a community is and don't need to ask or be told. A friend from the South sent me a newspaper clipping of a speech made in Kentucky by the writer Wendell Berry. Here is what he said: "By community, I mean . . . the indispensable form, intervening between public and private interests. The concerns of public and private, republic and citizen . . . are not adequate for the shaping of human life. Private life and public life, without the disciplines of community interest, necessarily gravitate toward competition and exploitation."

Community, then, is the "indispensable form" that intervenes between the individual (private interest) and government (public interest) to shape human life. Without it we "gravitate toward competition and exploitation."

Have we paid too little attention to the form that intervenes? Hospital care is a public matter. Because government pays, for Medicare and Medicaid patients, government regulates. At the same time, public policy dictates that to keep the cost down, hospitals must imitate the private sector and compete in the free market—with one another, with clinics, doctors' offices, outpatient centers—on the basis of quality, efficiency, price. Public policy has bypassed the community, jumped right over it to link up with the private sector, saying that market competition among hospitals will succeed where three decades of regulation have failed to hold down the cost of medical care. Market competition has not succeeded. The cost of medical care has gone up faster than any other part of the economy.

Medical care is a public matter, on the one hand, and a highly private one, on the other. Once during my early years in this hospital I asked Coleman to tell me about Art Seiler.

"Dr. Seiler is *my* doctor," Coleman said, speaking softly. "He's been my doctor for thirty years." Coleman said nothing more, and I knew I had stepped onto sacred ground. "My" doctor. The doctor to whom I am not a stranger, who has my history in his office files. Coleman could not talk about Art Seiler because he had not observed him in the way he observed the rest of the town and hospital, friends and acquaintances, so he did not have in his mind the common store of anecdotes about Dr. Seiler's comings and goings, the triumphs and losses of his daily routine. Coleman had observed none of these things. Nor had he heard the stories of the times Seiler laughed at his sick patients as he passed them in the hall and told them how ridiculous they looked, standing exposed and humiliated in the alcove outside the X ray department in gowns that cover the front but, alas, leave the back end hopelessly half tied with two thin strings. "God didn't bless us all with beautiful asses, did he? . . . Ha-ha-ha," he would shout down the corridor as he came toward them in a natty pair of red plaid trousers and a horse blanket of a jacket. Stories about him are everywhere. "Am I involved in *that?*" he asked one time, pointing at a tiny, ashen ninety-year-old lady lying wide-awake on a stretcher, his finger aimed directly at her nose. She stared up at him with eyes wide-open. The nurse pushing the stretcher said no, this was Mrs. Phillips, a patient of Dr. Anderson's. "Good," Dr. Seiler said, looking right at Mrs. Phillips. She had been a patient of his until last year. When Dr. Anderson came to town, she made a change.

Coleman repeated none of the stories about Art Seiler, to me or to anyone, because he had not heard them. The stories had been told in his presence, but he had not heard them. For Coleman the quintessential transaction of all health care—the doctor-patient relationship—was and is an inviolable trust on both sides. The doctor brings his best thinking and judgment to the condition of the patient, to achieve the best possible end result, *and* at the same time, the patient, through circumstance, places his trust in the doctor. The doctor, being so trusted, comes to trust the patient. And the patient becomes trustworthy. This is the relationship of Coleman Forbes and Art Seiler.

We treasure our private doctor-patient relationships, on the one hand, rail and cry out against the contradictions of public policy, on the other, and pay too little attention to the community at hand.

Now Mary Fuller, radiologic technologist, comes through the supper line, a textbook under her arm, and tells Flora that she prefers a table in the corner. Flora leads her to a large table in the center of the room where others are already seated, a noisy group of respiratory therapists and lab technologists and Vinnie, the pharmacist, all yakking it up in sprawled posture across table and chairs laughing at someone's crazy story, seemingly indifferent to the fact that they are on duty. But don't be fooled by the sight of them. People who work in small hospitals have a particular talent for straddling danger. At the first half syllable from the paging system announcing a code (a patient emergency, usually cardiac arrest) they are on their feet and gone, out of here, instant history, reassembled at a patient's side to pull him out of danger, then back to rearrange themselves in the same sprawl around the same table to pick up the story at the point where it was interrupted, without missing a beat. The story is usually about someone in some kind of spot, their having been in some themselves, but do not think they laugh at another person's predicament. They laugh with the humor of insiders.

I watch Mary Fuller defy Flora by walking to a table at the far end. She needs a few minutes of quiet, this small, serious woman who has worked a long day and is now covering the evening shift, who produces X-ray films without blur or fog, without artifacts or distortion, with good detail and contrast but not *too* good; if the film were too good, it might expose the patient to excess radiation. Mary strikes a professional balance between quality and danger. As far as I'm concerned, when it comes right down to it, she can sit at any table she likes. But Flora is agitated; no one has ever rejected her choice of table. The structure of her universe is suddenly shattered, and she raises her arms straight up over her head and howls in a high, shrill, piercing cry of pain, then turns and runs past the serving line and through the kitchen and out the back door, where she lies down in a wide pool of water in the emergency room driveway and will not move even when Vinnie and the lab techs and respiratory therapists surround her and tell her gently that she could be run over by an ambulance, then pick her up and ease her onto a stretcher in the emergency room, where Charlene Davis, nurse on duty, will observe her through the night.

Now in the cafeteria Dr. Talley shouts at Bev, "I'm going

with Miss Jannsen, get Seiler to cover," as he drops on the floor stacks of folders, charts, loose paper, the whole Kardex containing the daily working notations of nursing care, several of the folders scattering their contents of medical records in a wide swath under chairs and tables, the Kardex spinning out of control and Dr. Talley grabbing it by the roots of the cards themselves, ripping off pieces of corners and stuffing loose paper under his arm as he runs out the door to the ambulance, where the driver, Jim Boze, eases Miss Jannsen into the back for the trip to Portland.

Bev runs after him. "You can't take charts out of the hospital; it's a *rule.*"

"I'll stay with her, see you in a few days," Dr. Talley shouts back, and is gone. John Ferry, plant maintenance engineer, offers to chase the ambulance and bring back the charts. I watch him and his two assistants drive off in the van, past the window and out the driveway.

"Why does it take three guys to intercept an ambulance?" Bev asks. I haven't the faintest idea.

I stop by the emergency room to ask Dr. Anderson about Tim Bailey's visit this morning. Tim must be glad to be here, in shelter, out of that sudden April storm.

"The fire department can give Tim a cot for the night," I say.

"Tim is extremely ill," Dr. Anderson says. "His blood shows elevated enzymes. He could have a heart attack. I have admitted him for observation. Do you want him to die on the side of the road having just walked out of the hospital?"

"No."

"And Elizabeth Littlejohn is here. Her electrolytes are abnormal, and I will admit her because I don't like the look of her EKG. Besides, she is weak and depressed; apparently her grandfather threw her out of the house."

"Her unpaid account is seventy-six thousand dollars, we'll write it off, of course, but look, Dr. Anderson, are we doing her any good? I mean, what does she *need*?"

"She needs medical care. What did you think? Do you want

to put a three-legged stool here in the corner and sit on it and watch me practice medicine?"

"Yes. But not tonight."

It is late, time to go home.

FOUR

According to Coleman Forbes, the Littlejohn family lay heavily on Dr. Cage's mind. He referred to them in a letter he wrote during the Great Depression to the Committee on the Costs of Medical Care, whose final report, *Medical Care for the American People,* should have made a difference in hospitals. Coleman sends carbon copies of the letter to members of the strategic planning committee for background reading. The committee, Coleman says, will want to study the mistakes of the past before deciding on a plan for the future.

November 18, 1934

To the Distinguished Members of the Committee on the Costs of Medical Care

Dear Sirs:

Your survey of the health of the nation is the finest ever made, and it comes at a most urgent time. The serious economic depression we face together is threatening the very existence of our hospital.

I have read all twenty-eight volumes of your report, reading slowly and carefully (several volumes are quite long), and let me say right away that my admiration knows no limit. You have given us a definition of good medical care, something no one else has been able to do. The volumes line the bookcase in my study at home. Their good red leather bindings and gold stamping add an appearance of solid integrity to their length and number. I trust there are similar sets in the mahogany-paneled offices of the powerful members of our Congress. Perhaps you have delivered a set to President Roosevelt.

My question to you is this: What do we do now? Will your report sit on shelves and gather dust?

I have a proposal. If you have not already disbanded as a committee, you might consider it at your next conference.

My practice is in a small town on the coast of the rural state of Maine. In my professional solitude I have fallen into the poor habit of self-reflection, not good for a physician, but years of reflection on my decisions both right and wrong have forced me to expand my point of view. Your report speaks in words I could not find for myself but once on your pages are mine as if I had written them. I hope you will accept what I say as a compliment.

The authors of Volume No. 22, Drs. Lee and Jones (the latter is a Ph.D. but, even so, quite knowledgeable), have defined good medical care in unpretentious prose not given to false rhetoric, a pleasure to read. Best of all, they understand our situation.

Good medical care, they say, is limited to the practice of rational medicine based on the medical sciences. They speak the obvious, of course, but you must realize there are others, eclectics, naturists, chiropractors, cultists of all kinds in the rural counties and unorganized territories of my state, who treat with herbs and nostrums, manipulation and warm conversation.

Good medical care implies the application of modern scientific medicine to the needs of *all* the people. A profound statement, but how can we do this without intrusion by government? The latter is a stumbling block, particularly in Maine.

Good medical care emphasizes prevention. Drs. Lee and Jones say they detect a "trend" in medical practice from cure toward prevention. Vaccination, diet and daily elimination, care of women in the puerperal state, a periodic health examination for early diagnosis (some think I urge this for the fee I receive, and I spend precious time protesting their grossly insulting accusations, which hurt me deeply): These make the difference.

Good care is coordinated with social welfare work. Yesterday I visited the Littlejohn family, seven adults and five children living in a shack with a dirt floor and poor insulation. I treated the father, Lester, for tetanus infection and spasm of the respiratory muscles from a wound to his arm when he fell against the rusted blade of an old reaper and did not come to see me but let the wound fester for three days until his oldest boy, Mac, brought him in. I would admit him to the hospital except that he refuses to come. Then I examined his wife, Maureen, for bedsores; she does not move from her cot except to relieve herself in the hole outside. She is diabetic and must take her insulin and follow her diet. Mac's wife, Alma, is pregnant again, her sixth in six years. The four-year-old has scarlet fever and lies on his cot isolated only by an old wool blanket hanging halfway to the floor from the tar ceiling. I must have frequent urine specimens to watch for nephritis in this child, but the public health nurse cannot come every day. Lester's children lost all their teeth by the time they were twelve. None went to school. One daughter, Sula, is retarded and sits in the corner making a low sound like the mooing of a cow. I treat Mac for syphilis with arsenic and mercury compounds while instructing him in the need for character in staying away from infected women in Portland. Three days ago a fire broke out when the side of the wood stove fell onto the floor, but Sula doused it with water from the pump before any damage was done.

Good care treats the whole person, encourages a close and continuing personal relationship between physician and patient (yes, I strive for that, I have no family, only my patients), and, as you say, includes intelligent cooperation between the lay public and practitioners of scientific medicine. The latter is self-evident, but not everyone who is sick comes to the doctor's office, and not everyone who comes knows how to cooperate.

Or is your meaning a broader one? Are you asking the public to join the American Medical Association in opposing compulsory health insurance sponsored by government? That the public should be urged to vote against a Bolshevik system restricting the prerogatives of the medical profession is clear. But you see I am puzzled as to how we will achieve good medical care without aid from government. A grade school question: Isn't the government us?

And your final point. Good medical care coordinates all types of medical services.

To get what is needed—blood tests, the right kind of X rays, therapy following an injury—*you cannot imagine what it takes from here!* Long hours on the telephone to the larger hospitals, and often my calls do not go through, I talk only to the local operator and Central. Then I do not know from day to day whether the patient I send to Portland or Boston will have a long wait, a difficult trip in winter, or decide it is too hard to travel and forgo the test and treatment.

By your careful research you will have found solutions to this problem.

By your broad vision you are the most qualified to set standards for hospitals.

Now we come to my proposal. As a committee you must wrench the standardization of hospitals away from the American College of Surgeons. I have written to the College each year since 1918 asking for a survey of our hospital and have received no reply as the College chooses to ignore small hospitals in its race to steal the large ones for itself.

At some later date the College will recognize the value of small hospitals and include them in its standards. But you see, its standards will steer us in the wrong direction.

The standards apply to workshops for the convenience of surgeons: a separate medical staff excluding all but physicians to foster peer review and professional club gathering, adopt rules and policies, hold frequent meetings and refrain from the division of fees, establish handy laboratory and X-ray departments inside the hospital, and review complete case records on each patient containing important clinical data for (and I quote from the College's own *Bulletin* the words of their president) "observation for experiment, for making records, and for our own personal training."

So it was self-interest and a desire to take care of its own that prompted the College of Surgeons to set standards for hospitals, an effort it calls "a Great Movement in Civilization."

I, too, act with self-interest in my practice. For instance, when I suspected in a patient rheumatoid arthritis with underlying streptococcal infection, I sent a blood sample all the way to a laboratory in Boston at considerable expense to the patient, simply because I wanted to know the kind of infection. There is no treatment. No gain was to be made for the patient by this test. But I justified it by saying that such knowledge advances medicine and improves the larger human condition, and I carefully wrote in the record the results of the test, which were positive for hemolytic streptoccic agglutinins. The patient is a farmer, a gaunt man with grayish skin, not well-off, but he paid for the test in full by bringing us milk and fresh vegetables for several months so that the hospital trustees could account for the cost of the test through savings on food. His frequent trips to the hospital added to his fatigue. I did not tell him what I knew from the test results, and he did not ask me.

So I do not fault the American College of Surgeons on self-interest but rather on what it will do to our hospitals if allowed to continue. What good is a workshop for surgeons in the cycle of poverty and ignorance that surrounds us? There are dozens of families like the Littlejohns. Who will see to them if we do not? Who in these rural places will encourage the man who has gained a wooden leg but lost his nerve? Who will assist our old people who are chronically ill and live a long time without recovering? Every now and then, in the history of the world, a time comes when whole nations rise up and throw out the monstrous tyranny that oppresses them, giving power back to the people. Are we to allow a group of high-mouthed buffoons modeled after the Royal College of Surgeons in England (*England*, mind you, the very place our forefathers left behind, to find a better way in a new land) to take our hospitals down the road to disaster?

You must rescue the hospitals by substituting your key recommendation, the "health center," for the surgical workshop. Establish a health center in each town of over 15,000 population (at first we will appear too small to fit your arbitrary criteria, but we serve a large county).

Here is my plan: Our health center will be a consumer cooperative modeled after Dr. Michael Shadid's hospital in Elk City, Oklahoma, where farm families pay a monthly fee of 50 cents whether they are sick or well. This nation is full of ideas, even in the Southwest! Dr. Shadid has had the same experience I have: The poor stay home when they are ill rather than face the humiliation of having no means to pay; they come to him only after their wounds have festered, their infections spread to others, their diseases past the curable stages so that the cost of their care is greater.

All members of the cooperative will have a voice in the affairs of the hospital, causing chaos at first but in the end making known to one another our needs so that the *human* costs are contained. The managers of the shoe factory here want a plan to insure employees (and the company) against the ravaging cost of illness. The fishermen will join us, six trawlers are tied up, they cannot afford repairs and the men sit at home with their listless families. There is the farmers' Grange and the local milk cooperative run by churchwomen.

When our trustees approve the idea, we will begin. Two founders have died, and the board has replaced them with its own sons and nephews (it is a self-perpetuating board, you see, and the trustees interpret this literally), young people of a new enlightened generation bringing a new era of progress to our hospital.

In a health center, as you describe, the role of the family practitioner will be prominent and respected.

But the centerpiece of a health center is a group practice. I understand that, and I will be forced to invite another physician here. Does this mean my patients will choose between us, by preference? Some will go to the new doctor, thinking he has the answer I have not been able to find. But the new doctor will not know all I know about the patient. Much is captured in an elaborate system of record keeping we have developed here based on the End Result system of E. A. Codman, M.D., of whom you may have heard. But not all information is written down; some is sensory, from experience, from years of association that come forward when I see my patient. How will I convey the essence of a long doctor-patient relationship to a colleague who is a stranger?

Please answer me.

You say your recommendation for health centers will take years, decades, to "evolve." We do not have decades. We must act now.

You say that no group in America receives enough medical care because the nation spends only $30 per capita ($29 for personal care and $1 for public health). You say we must spend $36. An extraordinary finding. The average cost per patient day in general hospitals is already a startling $5! (In our hospital it is $3.11, but that is due to the cruel parsimony of the founding trustees.) You say we should spend more, and then, when we have won the battle against disease, dementia, ignorance, poverty, aging, war, pestilence, and a certain lack of interest in living, *then,* when we have achieved a better level of health, the cost of medical care will fall? Could you be wrong? (With all due respect to the distinguished and learned members of your committee.)

With mixed emotions I watch daily a crew under government pay building a new road inland from our town connecting to a brand-new paved highway stretching from Boston to Bangor. Several of my patients have found work with these crews of the public works projects. But the condition of medical care is far worse than the roads, and I wonder if President Roosevelt will consider it politically feasible now to introduce universal health insurance to the nation.

I await with eagerness your decision regarding the standardization of hospitals.

With gratitude and respect,
J. Cage, M.D.

Art Seiler writes on a sheet of paper: "I can't tell you what good medical care is, but I know it when I see it." He slips the sheet under the rubber band enclosing a stack of medical charts and pushes it across the meeting room table in my direction.

"How's that?"

Fortunately at this early hour of the morning the meeting room is empty, the air stale and safe, filled with life broth smells of coffee and cream of chipped beef in the cafeteria next door. It is May. Outside there is a haze of sunlight and a good land breeze. I can open the window a narrow half inch. Voices and a reassuring clatter of pans come from the kitchen behind the serving line.

Dr. Seiler and I have been over this ground so often it feels like home.

"Not quite explicit enough . . ."

Art Seiler knows better. He is playing a game. The game goes something like this: I will hold fast to the old collegial peer review—even though I know the world outside has changed—until you force me to do otherwise, and then, when mistakes happen in the new specific-criteria approach, when a patient suffers because of it, it will be *your* responsibility, not mine. . . .

When I am not around, he becomes himself, a conscientious man. From a distance I have watched him conduct a "utilization review," with four or five other physicians and two nurses around the table, considering seriously the cost to an insurance company of a procedure versus a patient's need for it: for a hip replacement, or an expensive MRI (magnetic resonance imaging) in Boston, or more days in the hospital. He can deal with cost and benefit.

Year after year Dr. Seiler's colleagues elect him president of the medical staff—"get Seiler," Dr. Talley and the others say in chorus, and he doesn't mind—and year after year he and I prepare for the coming of the Joint Commission. The last survey was three years ago. Accreditation by the Joint Commission is voluntary and highly desirable. Insurers look to it for evidence of quality.

". . . peer review among physicians, nothing to do with you, if we need you, we'll call you."

"The public wants hard facts on the results of medical care."

The American College of Surgeons wrote the standards for hospitals all by itself for thirty-four years, until 1951, when it invited others—the American College of Physicians, American Medical Association, American Hospital Association—to share the cumbersome territory by forming a Joint Commission on Accreditation of Hospitals (the word "Hospitals" has been changed to "Healthcare Organizations"). Until recently the Joint Commission relied on the "implicit" review of peers. As long as physicians of goodwill (honor bound to take care of their own colleagues) formed an organized medical staff, followed its bylaws, and gathered periodically to review one another's medical charts in a forum of their choosing, and as long as the records were reasonably complete, the medical staff met the standard for quality. And for many years the Joint Commission itself approached hospitals in the same way, in an agreeable spirit of educational partnership to guide them toward quality as a physician would take to the woodshed an erring colleague—a brother who knows only too well the unexplained failures and successes of both of them and knows that his colleague will not condemn him because there but for the grace of God goes he. In this warm rabbit hutch of professional empathy the public was often forgotten.

Recently serious problems of patient care at some accredited hospitals have changed the message coming from the Joint Commission.

The standards have grown in number and intensity—in sheer specificity—to fill 343 pages of a manual eight and one-half by eleven inches with twenty-eight chapters, appendices, an index, and a glossary of definitions for words like "indicator" ("measurement tool to monitor quality") and "practice guideline" ("standardized specification for care of the typical patient in the typical situation").

Some words from earlier manuals, such as "collegial" ("characterized by equal power and authority among peers"), have been struck from the new edition.

"You don't trust us," Dr. Seiler says.

"It's a matter of public trust, not private."

"Look, there is no way you can watch everyone all of the time. Even Big Brother can't do that."

"Not watch. More like sift—"

"Sift?"

"—care of the patient through a set of clinical indicators, as criteria of quality."

Some of the clinical indicators in the Joint Commission manual are quite specific. Dr. Seiler will ask for an example, and I know enough not to mention one of his own patients.

"Take Miss Jannsen, for instance, Dr. Talley's patient, a diagnosis of bronchogenic adenocarcinoma, primary, referred to Dr. Wing for a lobectomy. If he operates now in the early stage, her chances are good, but she refuses surgery, saying all she wants is to stay in her bed in room 20. Alternatives are radiation therapy—most patients die within the year—or chemotherapy, less useful. If untreated, she will die in six months or consent at the last minute to surgery, which will end up being a major procedure, a thoracotomy. This is poor-quality care because the simpler appropriate surgery was not done in the early stage, and there is nothing in the standards about a patient's preference, so all Dr. Talley can do is write down what she says and show that he tried to persuade her. . . ."

The Joint Commission surveyors—a physician, a nurse, a hospital administrator, all distinguished in their fields—rely on the written record. If elements of patient care are not documented, they did not occur. If they occurred, they would be written down. What is written down is what has occurred.

"You tread where you don't belong," Dr. Seiler tells me. "In the old days doctors handled these questions in private conversation."

To remind him again of the changes in store for medicine would be cruel bombardment of a man who has practiced hard and well within the confines of his profession and taken full advantage—who would not?—of medicine's privileged position, what Paul Starr, in his book *The Social Transformation of American Medicine,* calls, "one of the distinctive features of medical care in America . . . the access that private practition-

ers gained to hospitals, without becoming their employees."
Those who make the most vital decisions in the hospital are
not employed by it. I run the gamut from messenger to med-
dler, comrade to enemy, interpreter to antagonist. The bearer
of bad news is always in danger.

But the extraordinary thing is that hospitals have done
nothing to change this but instead have adapted chameleonlike
to the way the American College of Surgeons set hospital
standards in the first place. Accommodation and conciliation
have been our watchwords. Dr. Codman's End Result Idea was
in fact the catalyst for the founding of the American College of
Surgeons in 1913 and for the standardization of hospitals.
Then it quietly disappeared. It has taken us three quarters of a
century to return to it as a measure of hospital care. Where did
the idea hide? I believe that we who manage hospitals have
been cowardly not to bring it forward sooner but instead to
wait for something to happen, for monstrously bad patient
care to occur in accredited hospitals before the Joint Commission (mostly physicians) finally puts it to the page. Are we in
awe of medicine? Overworked, or merely lazy? Dependent
upon the presence of the right "incentives" before we act in the
interest of patients?

Part of it has to do with our training. In graduate schools of
business and management we studied, among other things, systems theory, which told us the following:

In a system a set of parts is united by a common purpose.
Every part is related to every other. Failure of a system can be
attributed to ignoring the relatedness of all parts. A systems
thinker states a common goal for all parts working together,
declares how each part works, defines relationships, provides
information, predicts outcomes, measures progress, modifies.
A sensible approach. But then the trouble starts. There are
two kinds of systems: closed and open. A closed system regulates itself. To manage a closed system is to assure self-
regulation, in preference to outside control. The latter
interferes with the system's natural internal order. When a
closed system is off course, a correction occurs, as when the
temperature of a room drops below the desired level and an

electric signal from the thermostat turns on the furnace to bring the temperature back up.

The thermostat regulates a closed system. But most social systems are open—that is, they interact frequently and intensely with their environment. A hospital is an open system. According to systems theory, its survival depends on its ability to adapt to its environment. To adapt, an open system exchanges information with the changing world around it. And the more information exchanged, the more difficult it is to control.

We have treated our medical staffs as if they were closed systems, subject to self-regulation, controlled from within. It was a lot easier for us.

"Those were gentlemanly times, Dr. Seiler, but private conversation among physicians sends no information to the public, which is paying, through government, and wants to know what it is paying for."

To achieve control in a complex open system, like a hospital, strong lines of feedback are essential. Norbert Wiener, the father of the science of feedback and control (called cybernetics, from the Greek word for "steersman"), defines "feedback" as "the control of a system by reinserting into the system the result of its performance." From feedback the system learns when it is not on course. To be on course is to be in a state of homeostasis, or harmony with one's environment.

We have no measure of the results of hospital care to insert into the system. We blame physicians for their closed system, but it is not physicians, it is we, in hospitals, who have lain low in a tortoiselike state of partial harmony—a well-deceived homeostasis. True, we have been around town seeking information for "marketing," which, as Tony says, is finding out what people want and finding a way to give it to them as long as that way is financially sound and holds the promise of a revenue flow. Much is made, in hospitals, of finding out what the community "needs." But it is our own survival that seems to matter to us more than anything else. *Survival*—in a form chosen for us by an elite group of surgeons early in the century. We have a closed system view of our own hospitals. Chameleonlike—as Rosemary Stevens describes us in her book

In Sickness and In Wealth—we lie low and adapt, draw information in but give little in return, not even to our own communities, about quality of hospital care. We let hearsay take care of it. A patient tells his or her friends what happened in the hospital, good or bad. Other than that, nothing; only the fact, or not, of accreditation by the Joint Commission. But the details of the survey are kept hidden in our files. We publish no objective evaluation of the care we provide. Are we afraid of telling the community the truth? The truth is good, for the most part. Mostly good care, a few mistakes. Will something less than perfection, if known, put us out of harmony with our environment? We behave as if a temporary loss of homeostasis were so unthinkable that it demanded letting the community think there is some mystery about medical care in hospitals, not to be discussed with our neighbors.

I think this is because we share with physicians more uncertainty than we care to admit. To establish a measure for the result of a hospital stay, we have to know the reason for the result. Often it is not clear exactly what the reason is: medical care itself or something else? And here again we were schooled in a model of medical care evaluation constructed by Avedis Donabedian, the most eloquent of the scholars of medical care organization. The Donabedian model has three parts: structure, process, and outcome. Structure refers to safe buildings and to organization: a board of trustees, a medical staff, managers and departments, qualified personnel, means of exchange (internal) of information. A good structure increases the *probability* of good performance.

Process is the set of activities that take place between practitioners and patients: examinations, tests, decisions, treatment. A good process, carefully thought out, increases the probability of a good result.

Structure and process indicate a potential for quality. Outcome, or the end result, is a measure of quality but with a caveat. What causes the outcome? To measure quality by outcome, we look for cause and effect. Certainty about the cause—a surgical procedure, a drug, a regimen of rest and prescribed diet, a set of exercises—requires information about the patient after he or she leaves the hospital. Does the patient follow instructions? Is the record complete? The list of intruders between cause and effect is long: genes of poor health, poverty, neglect, stress, forgotten instructions, grief and loss, the passage of time.

Donabedian makes this point: that process and outcome, as measures of quality, are interchangeable if certain conditions exist. If an element of process is established beyond a doubt as the cause of a favorable outcome, then the presence of that element is as good an indicator of quality as the outcome itself.

When we are sure of cause and effect, both process and outcome are indicators of good care. If there is doubt, then neither is valid.

The Joint Commission has stayed, until recently, in the comfortable land of structure and process where physicians can live with their uncertainty. Outcome is new territory.

There is no standard for community health, no measure of how a hospital looks beyond its walls.

Dr. Seiler postpones his morning rounds for a few more minutes to talk about the old days. This is for my benefit.

"In the old days I did what I pleased. I was director of the laboratory and chief of anesthesia, head of radiology, head of the emergency room, you name it. I was the one who decided whether a patient needed to see a specialist or not. The general practitioner commanded respect in those days, until the Joint Commission told the hospital to hire a specialist, an anesthesiologist, or forgo accreditation, that was it. The board took this dictum seriously and even tried to bribe me into taking on a partner. They thought that would bring in more patients and more fees, ha! to pay for specialists, and of course, specialists demand equipment, but I scared off every young doctor who came this way. . . ."

There is not much more we can do on the accreditation manual this morning.

"This is mild, Dr. Seiler, compared with what is coming. The results of explicit clinical indicators of patient care in this hospital will be entered into a national data base—"

"Forget it."

* * *

Gerry and Bev Tracey and I discuss Miss Janssen.

"I talked with her for an hour this morning," Bev says, "about the danger of letting a tumor like that go without surgery. The cancer could spread all through her body and she would die. Do you know what her answer was? 'I wasn't supposed to be born.' That's what she said."

"What did she mean?" Gerry asked.

"I don't know. She was so matter-of-fact. I told her that everyone who *was* born was *supposed* to be born, otherwise they wouldn't have been born, and who can say who is supposed to be born or not? But she said I didn't understand the facts. Her mother had a short bad marriage, and she, the baby, should not have happened, but in those days abortion was frowned on. Her mother was nice to her, but she, Miss Janssen, always knew she wasn't supposed to be around, so she could see no reason whatsoever to go to all this expense of surgery for somebody like her who isn't even supposed to be here in the first place, and why couldn't she stay right in her hospital bed, she will be no trouble."

"I suspect that's not the real reason," Gerry said. "She's afraid of surgery. Afraid of the pain."

"No, not the pain, she refused the pain injection last night and again this morning. I asked her why, and she said she doesn't mind pain because it lets her know she is really alive."

"What about Dr. Talley?"

"He gets the same answer," Bev says, "so what we need to do is go all out, with a *plan*. Like, one of us talks to her about how none of us is really *supposed* to be here, we all are more or less accidents but then not really, none of us would be here if we weren't welcome, know what I mean? Then we figure out how to persuade her, how to get *to* her, raise her self-esteem quotient, like what did she do—"

"She taught school."

"Okay, so we get school kids to visit, make a class project of her. Improve her self-image with all the kids pouring into her room with pictures, poems, dioramas, all that stuff. Then what? . . . Does she have a church?"

"She wrote down 'Catholic convert, lapsed.' "

"So we get Father O'Malley; the lapsed part doesn't bother him. Then the Auxiliary ladies, we turn them loose. . . ."

Gerry says, "She does have a right to refuse surgery if she wishes."

"But she *needs* it. . . ."

"If she refuses, we should find her a room in town. In someone's house," I say.

"On the ground floor," Gerry says.

FIVE

"Jack, for a hospital like ours there are two basic strategies. We can choose one or the other—"

"Only one way. Independence. That's what we fought for. While we were away fighting for freedom, there were some at home who were unfit, through no fault of their own, of course, but others . . . well, you have to think they were slackers dodging the draft, who stayed home and thought of ways to ruin the country."

Jack measures the century in clear terms: what happened before and what happened after the war. The war is World War II, and for him it was the marking event. Often he tries to engage Coleman or Tony or Art Seiler (they all were in the war) in reminiscence, but most of the time their attention is elsewhere. Tony imagines his own near future and longs to reconcile it with that of the nation. Art Seiler is engaged with the present—a good thing for his patients. Coleman's mind, though large, is taken up with finding its way out of the past before it is trapped there.

Jack and I are drafting the agenda for the next strategic planning committee meeting. We have moved chairs out to the lawn of the Shipley Wing to enjoy the first warm air of late May. He looks at me hard, as if he thinks my attention has wandered.

"Old Cage always wanted to hear what I had to say. When I came home from the war, he said I was of the new enlightened generation who had seen the world and as soon as I took my rightful place on our board, I would know how to reinvent the hospital to serve the people."

I am thinking, Who will take a rightful place on the board now? Soon Jack and others of his age will grow weary of this harsh enterprise. Soon there will be openings on the board for the new enlightened generation—the baby boomers, born after the war—who will know how to fix the health care system so that it serves the people.

"I, too, want to hear what you have to say."

"You see, before the war there was a lot of argument about health insurance, whether it should be voluntary or compulsory. Blue Cross was a voluntary plan that paid service benefits to groups of employed workers. Working people are worthy and upstanding, entitled to some benefit. Millett Barnstone owned the shoe factory in those days and wanted Blue Cross for his workers—"

We are in negotiations with the shoe factory now, over a new "preferred provider" arrangement. We compete with other hospitals, on the basis of cost and quality, to be the preferred provider for the factory's employees.

"—Blue Cross was a bulwark against government intrusion, preserving the vision of our Founding Fathers, who came to this new land for the right of self-determination. Cage said it was an idea from the Southwest, not New England, can you believe that? Started by Baylor Hospital in Texas to insure a group of schoolteachers, good citizens, and to assure payment to the hospital, that was its purpose. Maine signed on to Blue Cross in 1938, same year as the hurricane that blew the widow's walk clear off the roof of the old hospital, leaving a big hole. That night we had to plug the hole while the wind howled and the rain poured down in buckets. Uncle Mathias, Coleman Forbes, Tom Whitworth, and I held the four corners of a huge black tarpaulin up under the hole in the second-floor ceiling until Tom's son Donny could get there with plywood to nail it shut.

"Of course, this hospital didn't join the Blue Cross plan

that year, or the next three, it was busy with its own affairs, and then the war came."

Jack might like to know about Miss Jannsen, who, when I saw her this morning, was speaking about the war. She is back in the hospital. Dr. Talley admitted her for further evaluation and consultation with Dr. Wing about surgery. In the corridor she reached up from the stretcher and grabbed hold of my hand as Bev wheeled her down the hall. She was flushed and bright-eyed and chattering like a frightened robin.

"I am back, I am back! You're all here, just as I left you. I have my own pain now, my friends are here, I am back!"

Bev's hand rested on her shoulder. "You should rest, Miss Janssen, not talk."

"But I am talking to *you*. I must tell you about the war. I had no father or brother, no friends in the armed forces. My mother and I lived in a small apartment in Philadelphia, and we read the newspaper accounts of the war, every word. The closest the war came to us was the weekly air-raid practice in our building, when we turned out all the lights and went to a neighbor's apartment for apple cider. I wanted to join the war, but I could see no way to do so. A teacher at school liked my essays and took time to talk with me. I asked her what I could do for the war. She said I could pour the extra bacon fat from the pan into tin cans after breakfast—to make what? I wondered—and did I paste war stamps in a book that when full could be added to others and redeemed for a war bond? I had collected hundreds of stamps. I knitted scarves in khaki-colored yarn for soldiers. I wrote faithfully to my pen pal, a private in an artillery unit, but my letters were dull because I had little to say. I told the teacher about a newspaper story I read of a soldier who was shot in the stomach and lay under a tank for two days before he was found and another account of men at the Valley Forge Hospital whose faces had been disfigured. I didn't tell her the worst of what I read. It might have upset her. She was silent for a long time. Then she said: 'Imagine how it was, or is, for them. Use your imagination keenly and you will be there with them.' It was a serious answer. Young people seldom receive serious answers from adults, you know, and I held it like a precious gift. It was a secret way to join other human beings and be with them without having to travel. It was an end to loneliness. I worked hard on my new secret. When a classmate was injured, I practiced imagining the terrible pain of a sprained ankle or a twisted knee. When another classmate's mother died, I imagined how it would feel to have such a loss, and I cried to myself. Then I turned my new skill to the war. I lay on the ground with three soldiers who had been blown apart by a mine. I stood next to a sailor who knew that in just a few seconds he would drown. Together we could hear the roar of the water coming through the ship's portals. I felt fear when the water circled me and filled the hold until everything was dark. Every evening I read the newspaper and took myself to wherever I was needed by imagining the pain as if it were my own. Then the war ended. I grew older. My skill was well honed, I did not need to practice—"

"Bev, can I talk to you a minute?"

Bev did not look up at me. She was listening to Miss Janssen.

Jack continues.

". . . well, during the war there were Bolshevists in the Congress who wanted government control of hospitals. A few large hospitals would control the smaller ones, all tied together in a regional knot through universal health insurance. Under the guise of basic protection for the poor. And for the dissemination of medical knowledge. That's what they *said,* but that wasn't the reason: Control was what they wanted. Would have increased our taxes. Fortunately enough of us came home from the war in time to prevent it.

"Even in Maine there was a conspiracy, the Bingham Fund, it was called, to bring visiting specialists from the New England Medical Center to small hospitals. Cage made a case for it."

For a moment I am hopeful. "At the strategic planning committee meeting I will propose that we do exactly that—"

"Hmm . . . well, Cage pushed hard. Said it would be the perfect forum for exchange of information. Of course, we stopped it.

"But his craziest idea was a cooperative based on the farmers' Grange, useful, he said, for the mutual benefit of our neighbors, inexpensive and limited to direct service from this hospital, disbanding our responsible self-perpetuating board in favor of a citizen-elected hodgepodge. He said it was an idea from the Southwest. Then he would sigh, saying he wondered why New England was so tired. . . . Well, we sabotaged that one, too, by revealing it to be *contract* practice, as bad as the old days when doctors contracted for a prepaid fee to take care of groups of railroad workers and the like. No self-respecting physician would give up fee-for-service, although Cage said he wasn't so sure about that.

" 'Parts of the health system are related to other parts,' Cage said. What he wanted was to turn this into a health center with offices for himself and a dentist and public health nurses. 'Why aren't we an agent of the public health?' he would shout. I thought he had lost his mind. I said leave well enough alone, we've gotten by all these years, why change? We've also won a war; we must be doing something right."

Coleman told me that Dr. Cage and Jack always made time during the day to argue with each other.

He told me, too, that in the 1950s and 1960s, when a poor person of the town was admitted to the hospital, Jack interviewed the family. He received them in his office, gesturing to a row of ladder-back chairs, and questioned them about their income, their savings for a rainy day, and other means they might have to pay the hospital. If he already knew the people to be worthy and upstanding, he kept the interview short. But if they were of questionable character, or strangers, or if it were a person alone whom he knew to be lazy, out of work, drunk, bad-tempered, or a little crazy in the head, then he took more time, assumed a priestly role as he explained how generous men and women had made gifts to the hospital endowment for just this reason, to give charity care to those who could not pay. He told them that charity was the purest form of personal joy for those good donors and for himself. He never denied anyone. He simply savored the moment.

"Jack, do you remember Miss Jannsen? The patient Bev Tracey described during the March meeting of the strategic planning committee? Miss Janssen needs surgery but refuses it, and if she should change her mind later and consent, it will have to be a more radical procedure at this stage. Meanwhile, Dr. Talley will arrange other treatment for her, and it will cost us more than Medicare pays. We might pay for a room in town for her—"

Jack looked pleased. "Medicare is a fraud. I knew it. Set up to protect the elderly and the institutions that serve them, now it wants to destroy us all. The feds reneged on their bargain. Well, our endowment pays for charity but not for every stranger who wanders in here deciding for herself what she wants and doesn't want and making us victims of government fraud. She's not even one of our own."

"She is now."

"Well, in that case . . . we could argue it. Cage and I used to argue about the Littlejohn family. You know the Littlejohns?"

"Yes."

"Cage said they were the community's responsibility. But I knew they lacked will and self-discipline. Boys from around here drafted into the Army turned out to be in bad health. Cage said we could have been useful to the Littlejohns if we had been a different kind of hospital. Mac Littlejohn's three brothers were all anemic and couldn't read and had no teeth, but none of that kept them from induction. Mac's oldest daughter, Bess, was severely retarded, unable to dress herself, and sat on a barrel near her aunt Sula crying out in long, low-pitched, wailing sounds like the cow the Littlejohns kept tied to the rusted blade of a reaper behind the house. There were nine other children, ages fourteen down to three. Cage had a stack of file boxes filled with three-by-five cards all on the Littlejohns. You see, he wanted to know what treatments led to what kinds of end results, as he called them. Each month he instructed Mac's wife, Alma, in birth control methods, and she said she understood, but she was always pregnant, with complications, always, toxemia, high blood pressure, that kind of thing. He treated Mac's syphilis with a new drug called Bismarsen; it had one of the new miracle sulfa drugs in it. Mac took a job in the Bath shipyards, where on his second day he lifted heavy boxes from the freight cars to the platforms and strained his back so badly he could not walk; he had to lie still, listening to Bess and Sula. Alma could not remember to take her medicine for high blood pressure. None of the children went to school. One time Cage raised both arms and flung handfuls of white cards into the air. 'How can I know? It takes a *lifetime*!' he shouted. 'What kind of result? How soon? Information comes in pieces. A war intervenes.' I think he lost confidence in his own system."

I had imagined the white cards as an anchor for Dr. Cage. At least he could look back and see if a fact had been noted. The beginning of order. But beyond that he looked for cause and effect and found himself lost in a maze. What bears on what? And because he practiced alone, he came to believe that was the only way. All the information in one mind. His fear of another physician coming into his territory was a fear of losing access to information. More serious than the prospect of a lower income was not knowing what happened to the patient.

But to keep Jack on the path to a strategy for this hospital: This is my task. I may not be equal to it.

"Right after the war," he is saying, "coordination was a popular word. We heard about research firms combining their efforts. Get together, we were told, and you can produce something extraordinary, like penicillin. It was seductive, all right, sounded good in words, but we were smarter and kept our identity, at least until 1946, when we signed on to Blue Cross. The shoe factory demanded it, but it wasn't easy. It meant hiring another clerk to keep track of which hospital costs were 'allowable' and which were not. And it's been more clerks and more paperwork ever since.

"After the war Cage wrote letter after letter to the medical journals explaining the importance of national health insurance. Once we argued the whole night, sitting side by side on the horsehair sofa in the old hospital, about how to pay for medical care for the poor. Voluntary insurance will not pay for the unemployed, Cage said. He tried to tell me that our charitable care of the worthy poor was not the answer either. 'Everyone needs access to medical care,' he would shout, 'the worthy and unworthy rich, the worthy and unworthy poor, farmers, fishermen'—he pointed his finger at me, knowing my secretary paid her own hospital bills, our firm is too *small*, you see, to afford a Blue Cross plan—'wounded war veterans, children, the elderly, everyone.' I didn't disagree with him outright; one had to make allowances for an old man. 'Every civilized country in the *world* has a national health system,' he said. I refrained from detrimental remarks about other countries. Germany has had universal health insurance since 1883, but that hardly redeems the Germans, in my humble view. Besides, they had just lost a war.

"Cage said Blue Cross would take on an identity of its own, leaving the subscribers with no say in what it does. 'You watch,' he said, 'and why not deal with the government for universal health insurance right off the bat? At least it would be accountable to the sick and injured.' I didn't have a good answer to that, except to say that Cage wasn't right about everything."

If we could resurrect Dr. Cage from the dead and seat him in a chair at the meeting room table. . .

"Two basic strategies, Jack, as I see it: Either we join a hospital system or we stay by ourselves and become useful."

"Useful?" Jack looks confused.

"To our community, so it will keep us alive."

Jack says nothing, then: "Do you have it backwards? Should the community keep us alive so that we can be useful?"

With Jack around we may survive after all.

"In our own way, of course."

"Of course."

"Coleman, there are too many layers here, of old attitudes, choices made and buried."

"One thing at a time."

Coleman looks older, his face drawn.

"We're loners here," he says. "Apt to go our own way. Not inclined to give much thought to systems."

"How did we get into this fix?"

"It's the environment firing at us. Medicare, state regulators, all taking potshots."

"So we must be off course."

"No, just small. It's a challenge to hit small game. Like shooting quail."

"Coleman, if a system shows signs of breaking down, because of an overload, say, or a strain—"

"Trouble is, a system needs redundancy, and down heeyah in Maine we call that waste and duplication, can't afford that."

I should leave it there.

"Coleman, when a system encounters an obstacle in its path, and cannot maneuver around it without losing essential parts, what happens then?"

"What are you talking about?"

"The charitable mission of the hospital. The system keeps trying to go around it."

"Absorb it or blast it away."

I push one more question.

"So if a system has mislaid its purpose, and is full of holes, and worries too much about making peace with its environment . . . ?"

Coleman used to enjoy this kind of talk, but now he answers mechanically, as if we should move on.

"You are trying to fly on theory. Step onto the ground."

SIX

Buildings hold us to the ground and keep theorists at bay. We measure them by our own footsteps. When asked to describe our hospital, we tell you how many beds it has, how the interior space "flows," what parts of the building are old and crying out for renovation, and, most of all, what we plan to build in the near future. If we make a mistake in patient care, why, it is a problem of space—in the wrong shape, wrong size, located in the wrong part of the building.

Tony knows better. "Give me a nurse and a doctor, and I'll operate a hospital in a *tent*." Jack Mathias nods when Tony says this; it reminds him of the war.

Tony is ahead of his time. As for the rest of us, we keep on telling you about buildings.

It is early June—a moment in which to breathe. Lilacs are in bloom all over town. The air smells of a million years of ocean life. A harsh spring is behind us, and the onslaught of summer has not yet arrived. I will take this moment to tell you about the recent past and the buildings here. Fixed assets, we call them.

On the land where the old hospital stood before it was demolished in 1958 into a heap of shingles, floorboards, iron pipes, doorframes, and other perfectly salvageable items, three small redbrick buildings stand now in odd juxtaposition to one another. All are of red brick, but each is distinct in style. Each of the two oldest buildings reflects the personality of the individual trustee who husbanded its design and construction. The third is the work of a committee, a product of compromise.

The land is seven acres on the plateau of a hill between the town square and the river. Maple, oak, and sycamore trees, and one large elm, shade the ground and a corner of the 1958 building. The side of the hill slopes down to the river under a mass of low brush, left uncut. The river rises eleven feet from low tide to high. Your eye can measure it from a distance against the wooden pilings of the bridge that marks the river's end and the harbor's beginning.

The turn into the driveway is next to Chase's auto garage and leads up a steep incline past a brown shingle cottage (the old home for nurses), a new medical office building, and another small red cottage. Except for the manicured green lawn in front of the Shipley Wing, the land has been blackened to a fine asphalt surface on which yellow lines measure out parking spaces to the narrowest possible inch. What you see from the driveway is the gravel-topped flat roof of the 1958 building. Rusting metal slatted covers hold ventilators, air-handling units, other equipment. A squat brick facade hides the long, narrow T shape of the two-story building behind it. The 1958 building is forty-two feet wide and two hundred feet long, its front door bare to the weather, a utilitarian box lacking a single decorative gesture—no change of brick pattern from horizontal to vertical above or below the windows, no extra glass or extended roof, no arch, no column, no welcome. You could mistake it for the office side of a munitions factory.

"The architect was a local boy, gave us a good price," Jack told me. "His first big project. One long corridor was the most efficient design for a hospital, that's what he said. Seemed modern at the time."

Jack knows every brick and socket, every cinder block, chip of paint and plaster, its cost and utility.

By 1956 Jack and his board had raised more than $196,000 in donations. "It wasn't enough, so I told the architect to cut out everything he could. He took out most of the lobby but left room for four ladder-back chairs. Who wants to sit in a hospital lobby? And he took out the second elevator. One is plenty."

I had heard about the single elevator, from Bev Tracey: "When the elevator broke down, it was always at night or on the weekend, know what I mean? . . . So we put surgical patients on stretchers and wheeled them outside and around the back through a side door to get them into the operating room. The stairwell was too narrow, because you see with a *heavy* patient you need two people at the head and foot and then you need a third and fourth, one on each side of the stretcher. One evening Big Scotty Milliken, the lobsterman, went bad suddenly, and Dr. Seiler called for emergency surgery, but an hour before that the elevator stopped halfway between the first and ground floors and refused to budge. I was night supervisor and called the elevator company, and the repair crew was eighty miles away on another job. Scotty weighed in at three hundred pounds in those days and was doubled over in such pain that we couldn't walk him down the stairs, so we put him on a double stretcher of two stretchers tied together and covered him with blankets and wheeled him out the front door. Into fifteen inches of snow. Around the corner and down the steep path by the side of the building to the side door near the operating room. John Ferry shoveled ahead of us, then leaned his weight hard against the front of the stretcher as we eased Scotty feet first down the narrow strip. Beth slipped and let go of the stretcher, Sally and I held on, but the weight of it pulled us down and the stretcher began to roll, so John threw his full weight against it. Then John fell and rolled through the snow in front of the stretcher. Sally pulled herself up and grabbed Scotty under both arms and planted her feet in the unshoveled snow, which slowed the wheels to a stop against John, who was stretched out flat. I lay in the snow, holding the two back wheels. Beth got up and ran to get Dr. Seiler and Dr. Hart and the OR nurses, and we lifted Scotty and carried him on a human litter in through the side door to the operating room. John Ferry said it showed how well things work out if you roll along with them."

Jack had heard the story, too. Things like that are the exception, he said.

"We took out the second elevator, then the employees' lounge and the X-ray waiting room, narrowed the stairways and reduced the cafeteria by half, put beds in ward rooms, four to a room. Brought the cost down."

"So you applied for a federal grant?"

"Letting the government in . . . Hill-Burton was the beginning of federal and state control . . . it was the beginning of the end. Lost our independence and didn't even fight."

"We are still here, to decide our future."

The Hospital Survey and Construction Act of 1946, known as the Hill-Burton Act, was the first program to use federal funds for construction of voluntary not-for-profit hospitals. Its intent was to improve the health of the population through access to new or renovated hospitals, particularly in rural areas. States received the funds—$4.2 billion over twenty years—and allocated them according to a plan drawn up by each state, based on the number of inpatient beds per thousand population.

Hill-Burton made two requirements of its funded hospitals: Use the money for construction, and give free care to the poor who seek it. The act prohibited government interference into a community hospital's assumed right to determine its own policies. It was as if Congress had bent over backward not to infringe upon local autonomy. Writer and scholar Rosemary Stevens, in *American Medicine and the Public Interest*, calls it "a direct use of public money as a subsidy to make good the social deficiencies of private enterprise."

Jack said, "All we had to do, in exchange for the grant, was give free care to the poor. What we were doing anyway. In those days our free care was eight percent of expenses."

It is 11 percent now. It will take us belly-up.

"But there was a hidden catch," Jack said.

The hidden catch lay in the double message of the legislation. Hill-Burton made a statement: that a hospital made of bricks and mortar is a hospital; that its program or lack of program (no public health efforts, no ambulatory care) is not a factor; that the governing board's local judgment, and paternal attitude toward the poor, are to be preserved. On the other hand, a second message from Hill-Burton required regional planning for hospitals, by state, to assure access for all and avoid costly duplication. Planning implies that hospitals are parts of a system serving the whole. Planning requires some loss of autonomy.

A conflicting message within a single legislative act. Individual freedom versus regional planning. The double message of Hill-Burton set the tone for the turmoil in which hospitals operated for the next three decades.

Like most legislation, the Hill-Burton Act was passed as an alternative to other politically controversial proposals. National health insurance, for instance. Several times in this century it was almost enacted. It was a subject of Teddy Roosevelt's campaign in 1912. And it was originally written into the Social Security Act of 1935, but Franklin Roosevelt withdrew it when the American Medical Association threatened to oppose the entire bill if national health insurance was included. Harry Truman wanted national health insurance, but again the AMA opposed it as "regimentation and totalitarianism" and a threat to medical practice. Access to medical care for all, the AMA said, could be better achieved by building hospitals than by "socialized medicine." In the late 1940s most doctors at small community hospitals were members of the AMA. They supported bricks and mortar construction as an alternative to national health insurance.

"Then John Shipley stepped in—he was new in town then—and pledged the sixty-six-thousand-dollar difference. Of course, we elected him to the board right away."

"And then you could build."

"Then we could build, with local builders, of course, people we knew. Went smoothly because of that."

From the safety of hindsight, critics say that Hill-Burton directly increased the cost of hospital care by encouraging the building of too many inpatient beds. Supply creates demand; a hospital bed built is a hospital bed filled. In spite of efforts toward regional planning, too many inefficient and poorly run hospitals were allowed to exist. More wisely allocated funds might have gone to outpatient care, public health, and prevention. But without Hill-Burton this hospital and others like it, in rural or semirural communities and small towns, would not exist. Without hospitals rural communities would be without doctors. Few doctors want to practice in an isolated community where there is no hospital.

For almost three decades, until the early 1980s, regional planning was the favored national policy for controlling the rising cost of health care. The failure of planning had its roots in Hill-Burton. State plans were overridden by local voices and did little to encourage coordination among hospitals. Now regional planning is (temporarily, perhaps) out of fashion, considered less effective for controlling costs than market competition.

To Jack the 1958 building is still the "new hospital" that he and the others—congenial, like-minded, responsible men—planned together over lunches at Colligan's Inn, long meetings in the parlor of the old hospital, urgent discussions in the lobby of the bank, at the drugstore, in the corners of the school gymnasium before and after town meeting. Wherever they met they talked about the new hospital. Jack was the center of all of it. It took a lot of his time. But in a town like this one, time moves slowly and leaves open spaces. The hospital gives him a place to invest his loyalty.

"We cut the number of beds, then found that we didn't have enough. Then later, too many for acute care, not enough for long-term care, the next month the opposite—patients backed up in the halls, the emergency room—a month later, full circle back to empty beds again. How do you predict something like that?"

"It's difficult. You can only try."

John Shipley built the Shipley Wing during the 1960s. To say that he built it single-handedly would be close to the truth.

John Shipley is heir to a large industrial fortune created by his father. He is of the generation too young for the First and too old for the Second World War, of those who believe they missed the major events of their time. His inherited money allowed him to travel often to Rome and Paris and other centers of the artistic life he enjoyed and admired. Money gave him the leisure to try many things—painting, writing, study of languages—and to find himself on the outer edges of all of them, unable to penetrate the hard center, where the real work was being done by others. He came here to live in 1957. To his pleasure, his large gift to the hospital brought him immediate welcome and placed him at the center of the life of the town—a small center but a center nonetheless. He is a tall, solid man with a round pink face and squinting blue eyes. A shock of white hair stands out from his forehead. He wears a navy blue French beret, summer and winter, to acknowledge and make clear to all onlookers his connection with things artistic. When you speak to him, he looks at you and makes a decision (you can almost hear the discussion inside his head) whether or not to speak to you, to keep you for a brief moment unsure of your own next move. Then he speaks. In those days (Coleman told me) he wore knickers—loosely fitting trousers gathered into a cuff just below the knee, made of an iron-threaded tweed of British or Irish origin—and thick gray socks, a heavy tweed jacket with leather patches sewn onto each elbow, and he carried a gold-headed cane but never leaned on it, in those days.

At a cocktail party among the summer people John Shipley met the owners of the Sheltering Arms Nursing Home, eighteen miles west of here. The owners came often from New Jersey to check on their properties, mostly nursing homes in rural New England. They talked about the deep satisfaction, to them personally, of the nursing home business. Not only are the profits good, but there are rewards of a more spiritual nature in being part of a direct service industry instead of manufacturing some cold, lifeless product or sitting in a bank moving other people's money around. John remembered that pleasant conversation, and when his mother suffered a stroke, he brought her from a hospital in New York City straight to the Sheltering Arms, where he left her with a polite, quiet nurse. When he returned in a week to visit her, he found that she had been sitting on her bed all day. He rang the bell, but no one answered. He went to look for a nurse. In the living room there was a meeting in full progress of nurses and aides, coffee cups steaming. In the dining room he counted eighteen patients, alone except for one another, lined up along the walls in their wheelchairs, propped up and held secure by the trays fastened across the front and by straps that tied their arms securely to the backs of the chairs. Most were dozing, their heads lobbed to the side, mouths open. John found an empty wheelchair and brought it back to the room so that he could take his mother for a stroll away from the room and her roommate, an elderly lady lying on the bed, crying, "Quick, find them! Quick, find them, find them!" over and over. He leaned over the lady and spoke to her, but she stared through him with wide, empty eyes and kept on crying. He rang the bell again. The room was stuffy and smelled of urine, so he tried to open the window but found it stuck, unmovable, requiring a hammer and screwdriver to loosen the edges of the warped wooden frame. As he was helping his mother into the wheelchair, the polite nurse came quickly into the room. He asked if he could borrow a hammer and screwdriver to ease open the window. She interrupted him to say that the wheelchair was needed for another patient, and would he mind waiting a few minutes until the aides finished their meeting? John said nothing. He packed his mother's bag, put it in the car, picked his mother up in his arms, and drove her to his house, where she remained until the opening of the Shipley Wing.

According to Coleman, the sequence of events went something like this. John Shipley told the board the hospital should build a wing for long-term care of the elderly. It must be attached to the hospital, he said, to control the quality of care. If a patient needs a nurse or an aide and they are all lollygagging in some meeting, someone will come from the hospital side. And for a lab test or an X ray, a patient can be wheeled into the elevator and down the hall to the laboratory as a first stop and then on farther to radiology, then back up in the elevator to his or her room without going outside. Friends and relatives can walk over for a visit.

The board agreed. Everyone, even Jack Mathias, knew the need was there. Jack thought of the time when he would be too frail or disabled to live in his own house. It would be good never to have to go farther than this piece of hallowed ground.

"How will we pay for it?" asked Jack.

"The endowment, then a fund drive. I plan to make a substantial pledge myself."

"The endowment cannot be used," Jack said.

"Is it restricted?"

"No. It is for charitable care. If we spend it on a building, we won't have it."

The board voted to seek another Hill-Burton grant, begin a fund drive, and authorize John Shipley to engage an architect.

Meanwhile, Congress amended the Hill-Burton Act to strengthen local and regional planning among hospitals as a condition for construction grants. The new young director of the state Hill-Burton agency understood his charge: first, to be designated the "area-wide health planning agency" and obtain federal matching funds; after that, to assure cooperative planning between hospitals and government agencies. Each locality would write its own plan based on a process that local leaders would adopt after the young man had taught them how to do it. The local plan would nest congenially into a plan for the regional area and finally into a larger plan for the state. As a result, health services in the state would become cost effective, accessible to all, rationally distributed according to need. The young man's enthusiasm for the intellectual logic of public planning knew no bounds.

He gave John Shipley a hundred forms to fill out. John took the packet of forms and slid them along the surface of the meeting room table to Jack Mathias. Jack called his friend in the attorney general's office to find out what this was about. His friend assured him he would get the grant. The Hill-Burton agency is swamped. The young man wants to be sure he and his staff are selected as the area-wide planning agency. He is busy planning a strategy to keep his job. He is writing out his goals and objectives. He is assuring everybody a role in health planning. At least on paper. And that means everybody. Doctors, hospitals, town safety officers, the Environmental Protection Agency, housing authorities, public health nurses, police departments. And consumers. Most of all, consumers. With no axes to grind. He is up to his neck.

Jack was puzzled. Suppose the young bureaucrat and his staff were *not* "swamped" but comfortably established, their jobs secure, at least for the moment? What then? Could the hospital's project fail to meet a set of arbitrary criteria set up by a bureaucrat given too much power?

Maggie Healy in the business office filled out the forms. She read out loud, "Describe the local planning process."

"I'll take care of it," Jack said. And he did. He invited the town selectmen, the town clerk, and three other friends to lunch at Rick's. They took a big table in the middle of the room, and when others of the town came in, Jack invited them to join the table. When their food arrived, he brought up the subject of a new wing for a nursing home at the hospital and, if approved, how it would be there for them in the future should they ever need it. While they silently ate their lunch, he told them about the mother of a trustee who was in a nursing home where the windows were stuck and there was no ventilation in the room and all the nurses were in meetings and couldn't take her for a stroll in a wheelchair down the hall.

"That won't happen in our hospital," Jack told them.

"Sounds good," said the town clerk. Jack made a note of his comment.

"You gonna ask us for money, Jack?" Everyone laughed.

Jack went back to his office and dictated a page describing the meeting, to be put into the application as evidence of local planning.

John Shipley selected an architect and informed the board of his choice. He worked daily with his architect on the plans for his building.

The lawn in front of the Shipley Wing is wide, and the grass is of an even finer quality than the village green. In summer forsythia blooms at its edges. At the entrance there is a portico with two pairs of columns (made of brick, but columns nonetheless) supporting a pediment. Bunches of winterberry bushes grow at each side. Straight ahead, as you enter, is a large living room with a fireplace, a piano in the far left-hand corner, and over it, on the wall, three large paintings of rocks and the sea by John Shipley. Tall windows overlook the river beyond the slope of the hill. In summer the windows open easily. In winter, when the trees are bare and the brush is just a tangle of twigs and branches, you can see the pond formed by the river in one of its eddies and beyond that the two large fishing boats, one painted a brilliant red, the other dark green, tied between their moorings and the dark brown wooden pilings of the bridge. The light is good in the living room (and if John Shipley had had his way completely, the ceiling would have held a small round dome with a circular window set high at the apex, where sunlight would have dropped a beam straight down to the center of the blue-green carpet, and at night, at certain seasons, you would have been able to frame Orion's belt through the dome window if you had stood in a particular part of the room. That was his idea).

The Shipley Wing calls up an idea from an earlier time, of the hospital as a place where light and fresh air contribute to recovery. In pre–Civil War hospitals, poor environment—crowding, tainted air—was thought to be the cause of infection. A well-designed hospital was sited to enhance light and ventilation. Florence Nightingale, the English nurse who transformed hospital conditions and reorganized the training of nurses in the late nineteenth century, carried these ideas into a new definition of the role of the hospital: to provide an atmosphere in which the body can initiate and carry out its own healing process. Order, cleanliness, good nursing care, well-prepared food all contribute to the natural inclination of the body to heal itself of wound infection, dysentery, childbed fever, typhus. Long before general acceptance of the germ theory, long before sepsis became a standard procedure in surgery, before specialization in the medical profession, the holistic belief that environment contributes to healing was universal. Like a nineteenth-century pavilion hospital, the Shipley Wing is a single floor (with half basement) separate from other buildings to prevent cross infection, remote from disturbing influences, placed on landscaped grounds, with natural ventilation and maximum sunlight. A connecting corridor, through the basement, is a concession to modern efficiency.

"Why should it be separate?" Jack asked.

"So that patients with infectious diseases can be isolated from others," John Shipley replied.

"We have conquered infectious disease."

"Have we?"

Today a therapeutic environment is an amenity most modern hospitals cannot afford. Light is fluorescent; air is blown in through ducts. Convenience dictates the design of our buildings. We tend to locate services by their potential to produce revenue, resulting in an indeterminacy of design.

But how the decision was made to excavate only half a basement under the Shipley Wing is unclear from the record. The original design called for "shell space," excavated and left unfinished, its use to be decided later according to need. Jack liked the idea. It was a turning point, Coleman told me, for Jack to agree to spend money for something he could not see.

Every day that spring John Shipley walked the edge of the foundation of his building, pointing his cane at whatever luckless worker happened by. "You with the wheelbarrow. Your time is my money." He had pledged to meet the difference between the sum of grants and donations and the final building cost. Every wheelbarrow load slogging in the April mud meant more dollars from his pocket. Except that the dollars were pledged, not given. His pledge was carried as an asset on the hospital's balance sheet for twenty-five years. It is there today.

He watched the project fall behind schedule, by five, six, seven weeks. Snow and mud slowed it down. The snow was heavy; the ground stayed frozen; mud on top of the ground plagued the construction crew longer than usual. The project manager, John Ferry, showed him daily the work orders, bills of lading, materials ordered and on hand, detailed costs with freight charges, errors made and corrected, each worker's hourly wage with overtime. Together they made daily inspections, the two of them climbing down a makeshift ladder into the mud to examine the lines of the pit and measurements for the foundation. John Shipley enjoyed getting right down into the excavated cavity to see the shape of it. The bulldozer stopped when he entered the construction site and sat idle until he left.

"It never occurred to him," Coleman said, "that he ran up his own tab by the delays he created."

He studied each angle of the bulldozer's mud-covered target, leaned to the left and squinted, lining up the edges of the pit with the base of the 1958 building, leaned to the right and squinted again to line up the corner with the elm standing like an aged sentinel at the border of the hospital's land. He paced the pit that was to be the basement of the Shipley Wing, each step a consciously measured foot in length, then climbed out, walked to the telephone in the construction shack, and called Jack Mathias. He was stopping excavation immediately; half a basement was enough for any small hospital.

A mistake so obvious we never stop talking about it.

But by being a tyrant, John Shipley gave us an extraordinary building. Did he believe—does he now?—that a return to the old idea of a therapeutic environment would make a difference in health? He has an eye for form and function, an artist's eye. And he knew a good architect. But more than that, perhaps he has some deep understanding of what it means to be chronically ill. It was luck, of course. Only accidental good comes from a dictator who walks into a vacuum and does as he pleases. If the building had gone wrong, the hospital would have lived with its mistake for fifty, sixty, seventy years. By being small, we are at the mercy of whim and luck, according to who comes out of the blue and attaches to us—whom we allow, by the circumstances of the moment, to take over.

Systematic planning, on the other hand, with all parties involved, produces a practical, functional, even flexible hospital building. But not *this* building. I am drawn to the Shipley Wing, captivated by it. The board has permitted no changes to any part of it. The Shipley Wing is all of a piece, useful exactly as built. There is something whole and reassuring about that. We will never build anything like it again.

If you had stood on the flat gravel-covered roof of the 1958 building on a late August day in 1966, you would have seen long tables with white tablecloths on the lawn in front of the Shipley Wing and ladies in pink smocks preparing a punch bowl surrounded by platters of sandwiches and cakes. Then you could have turned and looked straight ahead into the window of the bank, where Jack Mathias, John Shipley, Art Seiler, and Coleman Forbes stood together in line for the teller. A blond pleasant-faced woman sat behind a card table near the door, where she could speak to everyone coming in or going out of the bank. On the table were stacks of pamphlets:

Amendments to the Social Security Act; Title 18, Medicare, a program of federal health insurance for all persons over sixty-five regardless of assets or income; *Title 19, Medicaid,* a combined federal-state program for care of the indigent.

Medicare and Medicaid, like Hill-Burton before them, were compromise responses to a half-century debate on national health insurance. The American Medical Association continued its opposition. In the 1950s the debate in Congress on health insurance shifted away from the universal and focused on two groups, the elderly and the indigent. Competing bills entered the fray. In 1958 the House Ways and Means Committee began public hearings on the Forand bill, to introduce hospital insurance for the elderly through Social Security. In 1960 Congress passed the Kerr-Mills Act providing federal grants to states for medical services to the needy elderly. Both Democrats and Republicans introduced bills to be studied, debated, opposed, and bargained through committees and subcommittees of the House and Senate. John F. Kennedy supported the King-Anderson bill, to provide both medical and hospital care to the elderly, regardless of financial need, through a compulsory tax. The AMA opposed King-Anderson and introduced its own plan, Eldercare, to assist needy elderly to purchase physicians' services through voluntary health insurance.

Finally, it was Wilbur Mills, chairman of the House Ways and Means Committee, who crafted the competing bills together. Health sociologist Odin W. Anderson, in *Health Services in the United States,* calls Medicare "a stunning symbol of the art of political compromise in this country." Medicare Part A, to pay for hospital and "extended care," kept the best features of the King-Anderson bill; Medicare Part B, to provide voluntary insurance for physician fees, came from the AMA Eldercare proposal. Medicaid, a federal-state program of health care for the poor, was a descendant of the Kerr-Mills bill.

For the signing of the Medicare bill in 1965, Lyndon Johnson chose the Truman Library in Independence, Missouri. Harry Truman was present at the signing.

"Independence," Jack Mathias said at the time. "Is that a joke? A joke on us."

Medicare and Medicaid were no longer a distant din in Washington. A Social Security representative had come to town in person and spoken directly to people in the bank lobby. The new legislation became local news. Now Coleman could run a story in the paper. He thought through the outlines of the story as he stood in line for the teller.

Art Seiler said a third-party payer would destroy the sacred doctor-patient relationship. A patient buys medical advice, something of value. He pays the doctor. If medical advice costs him money, he will follow it. If it is free, he will ignore it.

Jack wondered where to put another desk in the business office for extra help to handle Medicare and Medicaid claims. Could it go in the corner, behind Maggie? She might need two people to handle the new chart of accounts for cost finding, because Medicare was to pay hospital costs after the fact, in the manner of Blue Cross. Another ledger book, telephone line, new typewriter, file cabinet. A desk lamp. Costs money. Federal regulation costs too much.

John Shipley wondered if his mother would qualify for "extended care"—a level of nursing care more intense than a nursing home, less than a hospital. If so, Medicare would pay for her care in the Shipley Wing. Medicare would not pay for nursing home care.

The four men walked together across the town square and up the driveway to attend the Women's Auxiliary picnic on the lawn of the Shipley Wing. John looked pleased with his monument. Its timing was felicitous. Medicare will create a demand for hospital beds. Now we have them. Assign half the beds in the Shipley Wing for acute care, the other half for long-term care? Better yet, why not let the patient stay in the same bed and let the care itself *swing* from acute to long-term according to the patient's need? Then his mother would not have to move from building to building as her condition changed, not even down the hall. This makes good sense. Would a government program agree to it? These entitlements might have something in them after all.

"It's a *game*," Tony said. "Watch me."
"I'm watching."

"For outpatient space, put trailers on the front lawn of the Shipley Wing. Lease, not buy. Close together, you could fit as many as eight."

"*Trailers?* On the front lawn of the Shipley Wing?"

Tony is at his best when playing games. Except that he is already laughing at you before he is even well into the game because his mind has traveled around you twice and is circling back before you have caught the first turn. In his thirty-two years as chief executive of a large medical center in New York, he directed, guided, redesigned, shoved, and brought to successful conclusion dozens of building projects. The years from 1950 through the early 1980s were the expansion years of hospitals. Government grants through Hill-Burton, gifts from generous philanthropists, subsidies as part of Medicare reimbursement made possible towering new wings to be fitted onto the backs and sides of aging hospital buildings in the cities, and in the towns brand-new small hospitals sprang up where there had been only makeshift infirmaries in old houses. In those days inpatient care was the best care. Adding beds to a hospital was a sign of concern for one's community. It was Tony's heyday.

His idea of the trailers was not a curve; it was a serious proposal. Hospitals provide more and more outpatient care. Patients come in the morning for minor surgery—and for laboratory tests, X rays, EKGs—and leave the same day. Costs contained on the inpatient side bulge out in outpatient care. Tony and I used to argue.

"Tony, we need space."

"For what?"

"Well, for everything. For the emergency room. For outpatient surgery, physical therapy, chronic lung treatments. You talk about a cardiologist. What about the equipment that comes with him? Or her?"

"Well, what about it?"

"It needs *space.*"

He would look at me in silence, his face wrinkled in a half grin. "The key word is 'need,' " he would say, finally.

"*Trailers?* On the lawn of the Shipley Wing?" John Shipley was mystified. The other trustees were silent. It was a meeting of the executive committee of the board, Friday afternoon at five-thirty, scheduled regularly at that hour so that the new trustee, Skip Culbertson, could attend. Skip drives from Boston every weekend to the paradise, as he says, of his summer cottage by the ocean, where he and his beautiful family spend weekends and even winter over. It is more than worth it to us to hold board meetings on Fridays at that hour, to have him here. The world is no mystery to Skip. He knows it and loves it well. He knows the ways and means of large, complicated Boston hospitals, having served on their boards. Their din-filled labyrinth of internal political wars is transformed behind his handsome, kind face into worldly wisdom. Skip brings fresh air from the outside world. And he loves this small hospital. In board meetings he plays with it like a toy, lovingly, with full engagement. He is quiet while the local trustees have their full share of attention, gracious with the deeply perfect manners of America's aristocracy. Then when the discussion turns toward the edge of parochialism, or shortsightedness, he leans forward and holds back no longer.

"That is one option. But I want us to look carefully at the 1958 building. It has outlived its usefulness. The surgeons tell me it should be abandoned altogether."

"*Abandoned?*" asked Jack Mathias.

"Abandoned for patient care. I was talking to Sidney James at a cocktail party—he is a superb surgeon, and we are fortunate to have him here; we wouldn't want to lose him—and apparently the operating room is too small and on the wrong side of the building. It should be close to the intensive care unit. Surgical procedures require as much space in a small hospital as in a large one. We also need a room for ultrasound, which Dr. James says is a must for this hospital."

Jack cut off the discussion. "We cannot abandon the 1958 building. That is a given."

"We cannot put trailers in front of the Shipley Wing," said John Shipley. "That is a given."

Jack turned to me. "Bring us some alternatives."

One alternative was a new wing.

"Tony, we need a new wing."

Tony had another vision.

"The single community hospital will become as obsolete as the blacksmith. It will be absorbed into a system of medical way stations tied to a large hospital."

"Way stations?"

"Yes, for primary care and emergencies. With skilled nurses who fan out all over the town. A hospital without walls."

"When?"

"Not for decades. But expansion of hospitals is over. The skyrocketing cost of medical care has decided that. Think in terms of basic services."

"How will we compete if we think small and the nearby hospitals expand?"

"We will compete on price and quality."

"How?"

"That is for *you* to figure out," he said, laughing.

We used what we had. We carved up, renovated, patched, stretched, pushed, and provoked the 1958 building to the cracking point. But it didn't crack. Its resilience was extraordinary. We carefully examined every inside wall.

"Are you sure this is a retaining wall?" I asked John Ferry. "Can we cut out just eight and a half feet for a whirlpool bath in physical therapy? We are desperate."

"Do you want the roof to crash around your head?" he asked.

"Are you sure there is no other way to prop up the roof?"

John Ferry turned his head to the side, not willing to look straight in the eye of a person who knew so little about building construction. My ignorance shocked him. If I had to ask, then I couldn't be told. He will roll with any changes we want, within reason, but do not ask him if he is *sure* about a point of construction.

Then it was a matter of everyday comforts.

"Air-conditioning? In Maine?" asked Jack Mathias.

"Definitely. Hospital patients are sicker now. If a patient suffers heat prostration in July, the hospital is liable."

"New beds? What's wrong with the old ones?"

"The old ones grind up and down by means of a nurse winding a back-wrenching handle. *Impossible.* The new ones are all electric."

"But they cost nineteen hundred dollars apiece!"

"Yes, worth every penny. To compete in the hospital marketplace, we must keep up."

"We are here. Our competitors are elsewhere."

The fact that we are here ("If you are not very sick, you'll be fine at our local hospital, but if there is something really wrong, well, it's worth the long trip . . .") is one advantage. But access is not an element of quality. It is only a first step.

We compete for patients by adding new services. But which new services? Those that are profitable? Or those most needed by the people here? The two are not always the same.

At that time there was, as it happened, a mobile CAT scanner available to us—mobile by being installed on a large trailer truck, complete with technicians, prepared to travel great distances. "Studies show," Dr. James told me one late afternoon in the meeting room, "that even though these complex high-tech machines bounce all over the place on the washboard back roads of Maine, the quality of the scan is just as good as if the equipment were standing still in the radiology department of the Eastern Maine Medical Center in Bangor."

"How can that be? There aren't enough shock absorbers in the world to cushion a trailer on the road from Bangor to the coast."

Was there a catch? Yes. It was this: The owner of the mobile CAT scanner was American Medical International, a for-profit hospital company. The charges for tests were therefore high, to assure the firm a profit. Our patients, and their insurance companies, paid heavily for this convenience. In addition, to receive the trailer, we would have to cut a wide door and build a platform into the side of the building where the long side of the CAT scanner truck could connect by accordion-stretched extended walls so that patients were protected in snowstorms and bad weather.

"The charges for mobile CAT scans are high."

"So?"

"Well, it costs too much."

"Insurance will pay."

"It costs less to send a patient to Portland."

A weary but forbearing look crossed Dr. James's smooth face.

"Bring the mobile CAT scan here," he said in a quiet mock-pleading voice. "Just *do* it. It's convenient. And cheaper than the hospital's buying its own."

"We couldn't even consider buying our own."

"Well, there you are."

"Try not to confuse need with convenience," Tony suggested.

In the meantime, we ran out of space. John Ferry built a cinder-block partition down the middle of the old medical records room. We moved medical records to a section of the red cottage in order to put respiratory therapy in one half of the room and the EKG and treadmill in the other. Hospital departments are specialized. Each has a separate body of knowledge; each requires separate training, licensing, certification. Each requires a wall around it. John Ferry took the partition down and put it up again a few inches from where it had been, to make room for the extra ventilator in respiratory therapy requiring more space because of its wide wheelbase. John built a brick addition, 150 square feet, onto the outside wall of the laboratory to hold a multichannel analyzer, a beautiful machine that performs seventeen blood chemistry tests at once, giving a patient profile accurately and without delay, in time for the physician's morning rounds. The analyzer would share the new space with histology, where microscopic study of tissue can be done right here on the premises. One morning Dr. Somerville, pathologist, changed his mind. It would be more practical to send all histology to Bangor, where he and his friend from medical school had just invested in a joint for-profit laboratory venture that promised us fast turnaround time in return for a guarantee of all our business. It seems that Dr. Somerville had run into Dr. James and Skip Culbertson at a weekend cocktail party and worked out a different deal. The new lab space would not house the analyzer but would go to radiology, for ultrasound. What was the rest of the deal? I wondered. Something I don't know about? If I could get onto the cocktail circuit, I could cut off these end runs at the source with a convincing explanation of the value of a strategic plan.

I said, "We can put the analyzer in the front of the lab if we ask John Ferry to move the door fourteen inches."

"If you can't make it fit, then I will buy one with my own funds and open an office in town and run the tests myself," Dr. Somerville said. "Collecting, of course, all the fees. Every one of your doctors says he will refer all his tests to me if the hospital cannot provide for the needs of the laboratory."

Department managers measured their status according to numbers of square feet in their departments. At first they battled each other for space. Later they formed alliances, hatched plots and schemes, and presented them to me. Mary Fuller came with a joint delegation of radiology techs and operating room nurses: "If we could move the sterilizer in Central Sterile Supply down the side of the room just eight inches, then cut a door through to the main corridor, wall up the other side to make a reception area for Radiology, in return for which the recovery room gets the corner of room 2 in Radiology, in the back—that is, if we move the film processor to the other side of room 2 and cut through the back wall into Recovery to make room for one more stretcher—then Central Sterile Supply would get the little back dressing room in the operating room to use for cart storage, which would mean that the OR nurses would have to change their clothes in the supervisor's office, but she has agreed if . . ."

An employee showing ingenuity in making room for one more desk, stretcher, or treatment table was rewarded with smiles and a designation as Employee of the Month.

Jane Baker, physical therapist, came to see me: "The lab has a whole four hundred and eighty square feet of space and sees no patients. Aren't we here to take care of *patients*? Where is our whirlpool bath? Our rehab program? Do you know what Dr. Cage did, way back? He rented the *whole auto garage,* where he installed hot water and a hydrotherapy tub on one side, and on the other side he put disabled veterans to work teaching the newly disabled, first how to fix broken cars, then how to make shoes. From the shoe factory Dr. Cage borrowed dry-thread sewing and lasting machines, a machine for edge setting and wheeling and others for lacing and pulling over. He said an amputee is the best teacher for another amputee, a blind person for the blind. Blind, crippled, palsied, disfigured teachers taught the deaf, blind, burned, contorted, maimed, disfigured students, who came from farms and towns and fishing villages as far as thirty miles in a converted taxi that Donny Whitworth's father fixed up as a kind of bus. And there was a class in the construction of small wooden boats where they produced every year a twelve-foot dinghy which the entire group, all the students and the teachers, as many as twenty, and Donny Whitworth's father and Dr. Cage on a day in June would launch with the other dinghies made by previous classes and row on the river in a regular armada at a time of day chosen so that the people with arms could row efficiently, taking their passengers up the river with the tide coming in and back down the river to the town dock for a picnic with the tide going out. . . ."

Jane began to cry, and I wanted to promise her a brand-new building with everything in it.

"What the hospital offers, Jane, is you, with your skill. You are more than equipment and a building."

One late evening Jane waited at the hospital until the end of a board meeting at which I presented our Interim Interior Space Plan 14 with modest expenditures over and above the budget. Jane knew all the possible choices for Physical Therapy. We had discussed them for months. It could stay where it was in a room next to the lab (cramped and hard to find for the steady parade of elderly patients edging their way carefully into the building on walkers and in wheelchairs pushed by equally elderly companions). It could go into the old business cottage (worse, for elderly patients to climb an ice-slick path to the door, even with a new handrail). It could go into the Dietary storage room near the kitchen (large but subject to a serenade of kitchen sounds, pots and pans slamming into the sink, loud voices, deliveries wheeled through the hall). It could go into the back of the boiler room (if we moved Purchasing down into a basement cavern and cut windows and installed fire doors and plumbing).

Jane waited in the cafeteria until the trustees had left the meeting room and gone out into the snow-filled dark. She found in the wastebasket a copy of the interim interior space plan listing Physical Therapy's new location: the Dietary storage room. She borrowed a key from the nursing supervisor, Jessie Pace, and let herself in. Jessie found her an hour later sitting cross-legged in the middle of the room, carving the initials PT in the linoleum and pricking her finger so that drops of blood were etched in the carving. Around the initials she was building a model physical therapy department using boxes of strawberry Jell-O for stairs, cans of cling peaches for the whirlpool, and two rows of cylindrical paper towels balanced on cans of tuna fish to create parallel bars. Jessie put her arms around her and helped her to her feet. A light late-evening snow was rapidly turning into a blizzard. It was too late to drive home in so much snow. Jane took a folding cot to the Dietary storage room and slept like a baby the rest of the night.

A note from Tony appeared on my desk:

I have been talking with a brilliant young cardiologist, *brilliant*, I tell you, straight from a residency in Houston, Texas. I have advised him he can make a living here, considering the increase in the number of reasonably well-to-do residents, retired, whose lives are such a pleasure to them they would therefore like to extend them indefinitely and are now concerned about their hearts. Find space for a noninvasive cardiology lab. This is a market niche, an *opportunity*.

I telephoned Tony.

"Tony, do we *need* a cardiologist? The cost will escalate: trained cardiac technologists, monitoring systems, special equipment. And what about volume? Will there be enough volume to spread the costs, to assure quality? 'Need' is the key word, Tony. You told me that yourself."

Tony spoke slowly, with exasperation. "He will support his practice with high-revenue procedures. He is an expert in angioplasty, which, as you may know, is a much-perfected way of sending a small balloon on a catheter up through an artery to unblock the obstruction. It will be a *first* for a small hospital."

"Tony. The future. A medical way station. Shouldn't we become less sophisticated rather than more?"

"This is an opportunity. For quality."

Space was our common problem. The staff and I found an immediate rapport when we talked about space. I was comforted by the camaraderie of it, by having something to joke about. "Why, the EKG room is so small I put my toe in the door and the treadmill carried me out the back window and dumped me into the parking lot."

"Do you realize," Pete said, "that there is thirty-eight hundred square feet of unexcavated basement space under the Shipley Wing, left there to save *fifteen thousand dollars*?"

"Don't mention it. I feel sick when I think of it."

"How could a mistake like that happen?"

"The decision was made in April."

"Oh. Of course."

Lack of space was a red herring. It drew my mind away from other matters. Space is easy compared with quality.

On a late Friday evening we told the board that a vote against a new wing would be a vote for the Dark Ages—penury, cobwebs, and closing. Pete's numbers showed higher revenue with a new building. Gerry presented the danger (to patient care) of not building a wing with such drama and conviction that a vote against her would have been a vote against taking care of the sick. I praised the hospital as one with a long history of renewal, always with the good of the community in mind.

When the state licensing inspector made his unannounced tour of the hospital, he saw immediately, as we walked together past radiology, that the X-ray techs had quickly moved all the chairs out of the corridor (chairs in the corridor are a fire hazard; we could lose our license), piled them into a corner of the lower stairwell, and asked the patients to stand crowded together in the radiologist's office in their no-button gowns, looking like ghosts peering from a closet.

"Do you wish me to make your license contingent on submission of plans for a new building?" the inspector asked me.

"Yes."

The board voted to proceed. After four years of argument.

I knew I had mismanaged the project. Poor management is always the underlying factor. I had missed the point. It was more than the drying up of Hill-Burton, more than a reluctance to borrow money, or the harsh reminder of time passing in the obsolescence of the 1958 building that had been, only yesterday, the new hospital. The first point was obvious; I should have seen it. The trustees, with two exceptions, live in small houses and work in small offices. Any addition to a house is minimal, only what they absolutely need, nothing more. This has to do with the New England cold and the wasteful expense of heating extra space, but a larger part is modesty. If the chair is too big for the room, one looks for a smaller chair. The hospital, as an extension of themselves, should operate on the same principle. They heard neither the doctors' argument, that the hospital must spend to meet the growing complexity of medical care, nor mine, directed to achieving community confidence. My job was to persuade them to see other points of view, but what complicated it for me was a nagging notion, which grew stronger as I saw more of the wasteful extravagance of American health care, that their view had merit.

The second point was this: For me, managing the hospital is a job, the planning of a new building a project, a professional matter. But for the trustees, it is real life and as such needs attributes of lightness and richness, prolonged argument, weighing of pros and cons, getting together, agreeing and disagreeing. The project, to be lively, must stretch out. In a place defined by long gray weeks of winter cold followed by mud and frozen ground after which spring delays until finally it is hot for a short summer, in this place the project ran beyond its boundaries to fill the days and evenings of people who volunteer their time. To say it gave them something to do would simplify the truth too much. It gave them interest. It could not be hurried.

We began. Meetings with the architect and medical staff: "Must be large enough for future technology, do you want to stifle medical progress to save a few dollars?" Site plans, interior traffic studies, flow charts. Patient rooms should be on the quiet side of the building, away from ambulances. Not possible, with a triangular-shaped design that reduces the number of foot strides from nurse station to patient rooms. A roof overhang protects from sunlight glare in summer but lets in winter sun. Impossible, with a flat roof. Two elevators? Too expensive. Then stairways must be V-shaped, for stretchers. Not possible, that would cut into the lab. Birthing center and operating room must be on opposite sides of the building, to reduce infection; however, too great a distance between them prohibits common use of sterilizers. Medical records must be on doctors' line of travel to ensure timely completion of the medical chart.

"The exterior must frankly express the interior problems of hospital design," the architect said.

Cost estimate: "One hundred fifteen dollars per square foot, for what you need. This is the future, the cutting edge of medical care." The board fired the architect. The new architect (local) presented new drawings and cost figures: "One hundred three dollars per square foot, if we don't touch the present operating rooms." Dr. James and Dr. Wing scraped their chairs back from the table, left the meeting, and refused to talk further until we added a third operating room along with plans to expand the existing two.

"Why are you building this wing?" Coleman asked.

I was taken aback. Coleman had attended every board and committee meeting. We had gone over and over the need.

"I would put the money elsewhere if it were up to me."

"But we must keep up."

Hospitals of the 1980s achieved a state of harmony with their environment by increasing capacity. Besides, I would have been the laughingstock of my colleagues at other hospitals if I hadn't had a building program.

"If we have to build, build it right this time."

"What is right?"

"Build for the present, or build for a long future. Choose one or the other. Give the present the status it deserves, with prefabricated walls, designs that improve when changed around. Let future generations build something different, not tie their hands with the half-baked structures we throw up that will not melt away. Or take a different tack. What was built for us? Go into the cellars of the museum houses on the green and look at the wooden beams without turpentine, whole tree trunks, you can add anything to that center."

"Not fair, Coleman, to compare a hospital with an eighteenth-century house."

"I do not compare. I am talking about an act of kindness to the future. When it comes to buildings, we live in the Middle Ages. This new building. I suppose your architect is dutifully drawing a solid cement foundation and a pile of red brick on brick for each outside wall to form a box. And of course, cinder blocks for inside walls."

I said: "It is safe. Suppose we have an earthquake? And it is not a box. It has a rounded wall on the ground floor and a triangular patient care floor above. The most efficient design for a hospital. Seems modern."

"Like a turtle carrying a pyramid on its back. Or a seagoing red-eyed armadillo."

"Coleman, we cannot take time to reinvent the hospital."

"If we don't, who will? The big hospitals? Not likely. It must happen where new ideas are manageable. Someone must break the cycle of cost and debt and obsolescence."

I said: "It will have to be someone else. Look, there are people right now, in this place, who need a bed next to oxygen and a heart monitor within call of a nurse, who need surgery and recovery time and therapy. We must take care of them now. This building is connected to the old for continuity. We've trimmed the space and cost to the bone."

"And mortgaged the future to the bone."

The wing took five years to plan and one year to build. It is connected to the 1958 building on the southwest side. It cost $2.8 million. To build it, the hospital had to borrow money.

A Big Eight accounting firm guided us. First, a feasibility study. Project revenue over the next ten years. Did we project too optimistically? More patients than we could reasonably expect? Of course. To state that *fewer* patients would be admitted in the future would be to deny the necessity of the new building.

Big Eight showed the board how Medicare, Medicaid, and Blue Cross reimburse hospitals for capital costs (depreciation and interest) minus 15 percent on a complete new building once it is in use. Money flows into a hospital for depreciation of a new building. No money flows in for a building more than twenty years old.

"The nation would save money if hospital construction were slowed down," Coleman said in a meeting of the building committee.

"We can't worry about the nation, Coleman," Skip Culbertson said. "We have to take care of our own."

Raise $550,000 in donations, issue $1.5 million in tax-exempt revenue bonds, borrow $750,000 from Farmers Home at 5 percent.

"Farmers Home is a federal program; we want nothing to do with it," Jack Mathias said.

"We are already tied to the federal government through Hill-Burton and Medicare."

"Then stop taking Medicare patients."

"That's two thirds of our patients!"

"Do what Milo Hospital did. They got mad at Blue Cross and pulled out of the contract."

"But Milo is *closed*."

In accordance with the National Health Planning and Resources Administration Act of 1976 we applied for a certificate of need—the final teeth in regional planning to control capital expansion of hospitals. Without it we would receive no reimbursement from Medicare, Medicaid, or Blue Cross. Pete and I wrote the application, 177 pages of prose and numbers. (Is there that much to say about this hospital? Yes, and a lot more.) We presented it to the town planning board. No objection. A new hospital building means better medical care. We submitted it to the federal Health Systems Agency in Augusta.

It passed. We presented it in person to the state health commissioner.

"The building is lean," I explained, "no more than what we need. Note conservative plans for the operating room, only one new room and modest renovations to the other two because we are doing only a moderate amount of surgery."

That should interest the health bureaucrats of Maine, I thought. Studies (conducted in Maine by John Wennberg, M.D., of Dartmouth) show that too many surgical procedures in a small area, caused by physician uncertainty about whether to take the medical or surgical route, can be an indicator of poor quality.

"Never mind that," said the commissioner's chief planner. "How much of hospital endowment funds will you contribute to the building to reduce the cost of debt?"

Interest on hospital debt increases what the state pays for hospital care for Medicaid patients.

"Nothing."

"Nothing? It is common practice for a business to invest accumulated capital in its own renewal."

"The endowment fund is for charity care."

"Then your certificate of need is denied."

"War!" Jack Mathias shouted, back in the meeting room. "The state will destroy us. Our charitable mission stands in their way, they want to reduce us to rubble. I will not give up a penny of the endowment."

"A charitable organization can rebuild its base," Coleman said.

"Roll over and play dead, Coleman Forbes. Turn your back on the poor of our town."

"Our modern hospital will benefit the poor and the rich," said Skip Culbertson.

There was a long silence. I looked at Jack. His eyes narrowed, his shoulders went limp, his long arms hung loosely at his sides as he leaned so far back in his chair that the two front chair legs were off the floor in the air and the two back legs were balancing the weight of him. I wanted to cancel the whole project so this man would not have to endure another insult.

Does stubborn integrity count not at all? Is it old-fashioned to be tireless? To take frugal, unchanging care of an institution year after year so that it becomes a part of one's own body, so that every blow knocks against flesh? Seen through Jack's eyes—the state's feeble attempts at regional planning "to bring about a rational health care system" (system, indeed; all this talk about "systems," we are no more a health care system in this country than we are a confederacy of magicians)—the ruse is an outrage. The double messages are intolerable: Be charitable and competitive; be innovative and regulated; be compassionate and efficient; reduce your costs, provide access to everyone, give quality care. No wonder health care is in chaos.

Then Jack slammed the front legs of his chair on the floor and began his story.

"Ours, you see, was the Texas Division, but a lot of the men were not from Texas; they were from all over, Kansas and Tennessee and New Jersey, and a kid named Bart from Portsmouth, Rhode Island. We were in a place called Teano, in Italy. What I remember is climbing the side of a mountain on rough ground. Let me tell you, it was the rockiest mud-pit scrub ground I have ever seen, and the fog was so heavy I lost my direction and was hit in both legs. Two other guys were hit, too. We lay on the ground in a kind of circle for several days, eating the roots of bushes, living off whatever we could reach for on that land, catching rainwater in our hands. Then the aidmen brought us in on mules to the evacuation hospital, which was a tent with a dirt floor that stayed pretty dry although it rained most days. Outside, the mud was deep, and a nurse got stuck in it up to her knees. It took two men to pull her out.

"Well, the tent was about the size of the fish house on our town dock and was held up in the center by a metal pole, so we slept with our heads to the center, no space between our litters. The way the guys who ran the place made do with not much was really amazing when I think of how Uncle Mathias used to talk about making do with what you have. The nurses rigged up a desk at the side of the tent with nothing but Italian cinder blocks holding up a wooden crate turned sideways to make shelves for medicines and support the lid of the crate, which rested at the other end on the nurse's lap so she could write in the medical record. There was a bare light bulb hanging from the top of the tent. Someone said the first thing these guys got hold of was a generator. By the way, is our old generator working? Suppose the lights go out?"

"John Ferry tests it daily."

"Ah. Well, the fellow lying next to me was Bart, from Portsmouth, Rhode Island. He cried a lot, but in the fighting he was brave. Before I was hit, we crossed this river called the Rapido; it means 'fast' in Italian, and it had a fast current like our river, only no tide. We crossed at night under German artillery fire from high on the slope of a mountain called Monte Cassino, where the Germans had been dug in for months. Bart ran through the minefield to grab hold of a man whose side had been blown through by a land mine. He grabbed him under the shoulders and hauled him along to the boats we had hidden, got him into a boat, and was lucky because a lot of the boats were full of shell holes. I saw him launch and reach the other side of the river, only about fifty feet away, but the mudbank on that side was slippery and steep, so he couldn't pull him up. That was where I had to leave him and go on."

Jack stopped, as if remembering something he thought he could have done differently. Then he continued.

"Bart was hit, and the two of them lay unconscious in the dark by the river, and when he woke up, the man was gone. He looked for him in the river. The man must have drowned and been washed downstream. But what he cried about in the hospital tent was an old monastery called Monte Cassino, the same name as the mountain, founded by St. Benedict in the sixth century. Bart said that Benedict was the first to write in the code of rules of a monastery that it will have a hospital for charitable care of the sick. You see, Bart went to a Benedictine school at home and knew a lot about it. The mountain and the monastery were strategically in the way of the Allies' progress in the war. We thought the Germans were occupying the monastery itself, so our own B-26s dropped several hundred tons of bombs on the abbey, and it was a smoking rubble. A lot of people thought bombing the abbey was a good idea, but Bart said there were no Germans in it, nobody in it but refugees and sick people. I don't know how he knew that, but I felt bad for him, so I said worse things had happened in the war and were happening at that moment, but that was the wrong thing to say because it made him cry harder and shake all over. Worse is not the point, he shouted: It doesn't matter what is worse when we bomb the bejesus out of the beginning of Western charity because it is in the way, we, the Allies, were sent there in the first place to preserve a civilization, not destroy it, and he was heaving and shaking so hard that I pulled myself up and fell across his back to keep him from hitting his head over and over on the metal pole. The nurse told me we would bomb the monastery again the next day—she listened to the radio a lot and talked to the officers—but I said nothing about it to Bart."

Jack leaned forward with his upper body stretched across the table and stayed there for a few seconds. It seemed like an eternity.

"Tony, it's time for you to become involved."

"Can't handle it, eh?"

"In Maine we use what we have. I have you."

"What do you expect *me* to do?"

"You are a statesman, Tony. You always know what is important. Whether you act on your knowledge or not is something else. Most of us do not. A hospital without walls, you say? We all talk theory to each other as balm to the spirit. If everyone would stop being sick for six months, then we could turn theory to practice and reinvent the hospital, but we are caught in a vortex of need and pressure, of demand for specialists and rooms full of miraculous gadgets to go with them. We know the cost, but our hands are tied; we have to survive."

Two days later the board voted to transfer $300,000 from the Endowment Fund to the Building Fund. The commissioner of health noted the transfer and issued a certificate of need. Jack said we had allowed the state to fool us into destroying our charitable mission without a fight.

Next, the bonds. An army entered the meeting room: the state Municipal Bond Authority, Wall Street underwriter for the bonds, Big Eight, Farmers Home Administration, counsel for the hospital, counsel for the underwriter, counsel for the bond authority, bond counsel.

"Who *are* those guys?" asked Dr. Seiler, passing us in the hall on our way to the meeting room.

"Suits from New York," Bev Tracey said, going the other way. Dark gray suits, striped Ivy ties, click of good leather briefcases opening and shutting, talk of airline schedules and ways to arrange a weekend stopover in Nantucket. The Farmers Home bureaucrat from Augusta looked shabby in his thin greenish jacket and brown trousers. Did we all look shabby? I thought about it briefly. The interest on the bonds was 12 percent.

"Highway robbery. We are mortgaging the health of our neighbors," said Jack Mathias.

"We can refinance when interest rates drop."

"Can you guarantee they will drop?"

"No."

"Then we won't build. That young man from Wall Street called these junk bonds. He thought I couldn't hear him, but I heard him all right."

Later in the same week Mr. Caleb, a widower and newcomer to the town—a charming man who had traveled extensively in Europe until a few weeks before, when he returned to New England and bought a spacious old shingled house on the upper Coast Road—called Jack Mathias to offer a gift of one-half million dollars to the hospital's fund-raising campaign. Right away Jack drew him into the center by inviting him to join the hospital's board of trustees.

We sent bid documents to construction firms.

"We want a construction firm from here," Jack said.

Silence. I waited a century before I spoke.

"By law, on a project using federal funds, we have to take the low bidder."

"But the low bidder is *not from Maine,*" Jack said.

Gradually hospital boards will replace the Jack Mathiases. Who will take their places? Young corporate planners, systems engineers, strategic thinkers who have memories as enduring as a snowflake. All to the good, of course. To survive as a small hospital, we must be "fantastically innovative," as economist Eli Ginzberg has advised us. But who will be loyal?

I looked at Tony, who avoided my gaze by turning to study

the spines of the bound volumes of the *New England Journal of Medicine* stacked along the shelf behind his head. I looked at Coleman, seated at the far end of the table. You already know what I think, his noncommittal stare told me. Skip sat quietly. The architect left the room. I walked casually over to the window to watch the ambulance pulling in at the emergency room door. If I look hard enough, I thought, I might be able to see exactly who that is being wheeled in on a stretcher. Pete got up and headed for the cafeteria to refill his coffee cup. We can stop the building now. Or is it too late? If we do, we will lose the doctors' confidence. They will drift away to modern hospitals. We will lose the confidence of our employees, especially nurses, who are now in short supply and can work in any hospital they choose.

Refuse to take the low bidder? Lose the Farmers Home loan at 5 percent, borrow another $750,000 through municipal bonds at 12 percent? We can't afford it.

"Whom do you trust the most in this town?" I asked Jack.

"Trust? Well, lots of people. All the old-timers."

"I mean, with construction."

"John Ferry."

"We'll hire John Ferry as clerk of the works for the building. He will count pennies and bricks, measure every inch of cement, watch for quality. Nothing gets by him."

We were under construction. What we wanted most was to see the roof go up before the snow began.

Soon we would have enough space, for the time being, and the red herring would disappear to be replaced by other problems, diverse and complicated, ones you cannot easily set up for display and rally everyone around.

SEVEN

Summer. The lilacs have bloomed; the maple trees are a deep green. The river is dotted with boats moored on both sides of the channel. Already in the second week of August the early-morning air is cold, signaling the coming of autumn. Summer is a short season here, never leisurely. From early June to late August the town is filled with tourists. Hundreds of tourists. Most come in cars. Some arrive in buses that are taller than the tallest building on the green except for the Congregational church.

This flood of cars and buses is what the people here prepare for all winter, but when it comes, it always surprises them, as if it had never happened before.

"Never seen anything like it," Father O'Malley said to me yesterday in the Shipley Wing.

I see a lot of Father O'Malley. Five years ago he came as priest to St. Christopher's parish—he is new in town, newer than I am—a man of sixty or so with gray hair and a modest bespectacled look, preoccupied but not unobservant, tired but not excessively so and not bored. He is in the hospital several times a day, not because we ask him to be or because he has that many parishioners who are patients. Nor does he appear to be seeking converts to Catholicism. He is simply here, summer and winter, as if he has always been here but has not yet discovered all there is to discover. This is a Protestant town that happens to have a Catholic church, but in the hospital it is Father O'Malley who at any time of day walks through the halls, breaking up despair like a ship cutting through Arctic ice, who turns the corner of a corridor as naturally as a handrail and enters with ease a conversation or a vigil. With the Protestant ministers—fine men well organized among themselves to cover the hospital—the schedule is the guide: "I'll be there at four forty-five," or "The Reverend Welch is taking call today." Whenever I see Father O'Malley, he is on his way somewhere, but I never see him going out nor do I see him coming in. He appears suddenly as if out of the air.

"More than last summer?"

"Oh my, yes, many more."

The summer people, those who own cottages here, also complain about the tourists.

"I have never seen anything like it," says Mrs. Butterworth on her way to a meeting of the Summer Ladies Committee. "I could not make a left turn. There is nowhere to park. The town was simply not designed for this *onslaught.*"

Art Seiler shouts, "A host of tourists, some of them sick!" as he bounces lightly on his feet along the corridor.

I have been curious about how, years ago, Dr. Cage took the news that the young Arthur Seiler, M.D., had come to practice here. I asked Coleman.

"Resent it? He never said a word. One night, it was June 1959, Dr. Cage died in his sleep. No one even knew he had been ill. When he did not come to the hospital for morning rounds, Jack and Tom Whitworth and I went to the house and knocked and finally broke the back windowpane. We found him upstairs in his bed, lights blazing, the bed and floor strewn with journals. He had died in no pain, we thought, and Dr. Seiler came immediately and confirmed death from heart failure. The ambulance volunteers carried him down the narrow stairs of his house. It required three of them to ease that large man down without breaking a rail in the banister and out through his office waiting room through the low, narrow doorway to the lane, where two of his elderly patients were already waiting for the office to open. Seiler was magnificent, spoke to

them both, saying Dr. Cage had just died and they might want
to consider starting in with a new doctor, and gave each one
his card, offering to see them in his office in the next hour. In
fact, Cage's bare feet were barely out the front door before
Seiler had all of his patient records neatly piled up to take to
his office, where he kept them under lock and key until patients made appointments with him to ask for them. . . ."

Often on late-summer afternoons Art Seiler switches his
telephone so that it rings in the hospital emergency room,
closes his office, and ten minutes later is on his dock on the
river, starting up his big white cigarette boat. He throws off the
ropes and steers slowly down the river to the treacherous entrance to the harbor, where the current doubles back on you,
around the bell buoy to the open ocean, then back, joining the
lobstermen returning to the harbor with the evening's catch.
He knows all the lobstermen and the crews of the two large
fishing boats. Often on these summer evenings Big Scotty
Milliken waits for him. Then the two of them steer out
through the harbor together, one boat ahead of the other. Most
of the lobster pots in the harbor belong to Big Scotty. You can
tell they are his by the bright blue and yellow painted markers
bobbing above the surface, an unseen rope connected to the
square cagelike pots lying on the ocean floor. The markers of
the other lobstermen are of different colors—some white with
a red circle, some dark green or black, many combinations.
Scotty's boat is not the biggest in the harbor, but it is sturdy
and well kept, always in good working order. The hull is
painted white with a narrow blue and yellow stripe near the
waterline. Scotty paints it every year in late March—hauls it
onto the riverbank, scrubs the barnacles and seaweed off the
bottom.

Scotty still weighs a good three hundred pounds dry. He has
a dark beard and a big, bellowing voice. In his black rubber
jacket and yellow slicker apron he is a noticeable figure, the
unstated emperor of the harbor in lobster season. You can see
him around five-thirty in the morning guiding his boat through
the early mist, under the bridge—he moors upriver, near Art
Seiler's dock—and out of the harbor with such ease that he appears to be doing nothing, as if the boat had memorized the

way long ago. He hooks his traps and hauls them to the deck to retrieve the catch and replenish the bait before dropping them back, then returns to his mooring by eight. The rest of the day Scotty drives the ambulance for the Volunteer Ambulance Association. In late afternoon he repeats his rounds for the day's catch.

Scotty and Art Seiler converse back and forth. The water carries voices. They talk in normal tones and hear each other perfectly. In the summer evening light, the cool ocean air beginning to touch the harbor, others call to them, and from Boston Whalers the teenage children of the summer people call, "Hey, Dr. Seiler, what a great boat!" and the Yacht Club summer sailors wave from their 210s. Slowly the numbers swell, the sailboats moving without motor. A tourist in a rented motorboat cuts his speed to lower the height and force of his wake.

If you could pull back and watch from a high place (or ride the wings of a sea gull), you would see at this hour a little armada with Art Seiler at the center surrounded by summer children so at ease in these waters, as at home in their Whalers and sailboats as the lobstermen are in their sturdy craft. The good manners of the lobstermen and summer children are complete; it never occurs to them to make even the slightest signal that he is anything other than a great sailor himself or shows anything but skill in guiding his boat through strong currents and unexpected side washes. Three times in the past he has collided with another boat, and once he tangled with two lobster pot lines at once. But these incidents are forgotten. The summer sailors are so polite they do not offer to guide you, but if you are not one of them, they simply sail alongside you, hovering and watching out but not obviously so, ready to help.

This evening the unexpected happened. Dr. Seiler fell out of his boat. It was a freak accident, a combination of sudden high wind and turning current along with an unusually strong wake created by a young teenager, a stranger—not from here, not of the summer colony, not recognized by anyone who was there—who came suddenly out of nowhere in a motorboat too close and too fast and tipped Art Seiler's boat so far to the port side that he lost his balance and went in chest first with his arms flung wide. Big Scotty roared like a bull as he turned his boat around to be the first to throw a rope to Art Seiler, who was flailing and bobbing among the blue and yellow markers and who reached for the rope but missed it, the current carrying him this way and that in an eddy of tidal backwash dangerously close to the rocks. Scotty put his boat in neutral and jumped into the water with the rope in one hand and grabbed Seiler by the neck with the other and held on to him in the rough, choppy water until the summer sailors could maneuver close enough—"*Took* them a few minutes," Donny Whitworth said—and two of them together in a small Whaler could pull both Seiler and Scotty out of the water and then move quickly to pull up alongside Scotty's boat, where one of them boarded and steered it away from the rocks just in time. The incoming tide washed Seiler's boat into the channel, where it headed rudderless toward the shoals at the edge of the harbor and gave the summer sailors a chase, but they caught it, too, after a few minutes and a lot of shouting of instructions back and forth.

This evening the little armada held close ranks as it approached the narrow entrance to the harbor. The summer sailors waved, and the lobstermen waved back, friendlier than usual. Several of the summer sailors docked at the Yacht Club. The lobstermen pulled alongside the town dock to deliver their catch, then caught their moorings to settle the boats and climb into dinghies to row for shore and home. Scotty pulled in at the town dock and called to the driver of a truck waiting to pack and load his lobsters. Art Seiler waved and kept going, turning left up the river, the brilliant light beginning to fade as he tied his boat to the dock and unloaded his gear. He thought he'd wait there for Scotty, to thank him one more time for saving his life.

In summer the tourists who stay more than a few hours fill the offering plates of the local churches on Sunday, eat lunch at Rick's (All Seasons), buy gasoline at Cumberland Farms, film at the Rite-Aid pharmacy, and have their hair cut at Dick's Barber Shop. Lucky ones stay a few days, at the Inn at Harmon Park or Dockside. Some become ill and are admitted to the hospital. This evening the hospital is full. All beds are taken, and the emergency room is backed up with six urgent cases and fourteen less urgent. I consider issuing a "divert" to the outlying rescue squads, to let them know we are full until further notice, but decide against it. Dr. Anderson is on duty in the emergency room. He is more than competent. Three doctors are on call, for backup. We will put temporary beds in the meeting room if necessary.

The emergency waiting area seems a gallery of wax figures staring straight ahead or down at the floor, uneasy in their patience, too quiet. Their eyes dart up expectantly when I walk in and slowly return to a lowered stare when they see I am neither a doctor nor a nurse. Many are tourists, uncertain of how they will be treated in this small, unfamiliar hospital. What are the signs of quality here? How do I let them know their chances are good? I sit down to rest in the one empty place, the center brown vinyl cushion on a three-seat sofa. What would I think, sitting here, if I were a stranger? What can I say to them? Charlene Davis is the nurse on duty. I am comfortable, knowing her competence, but these others have no access to my secret knowledge. For them it is like waiting in a cave without knowing how long the wait will be or who will come at the end of it. The absence of light in the corridor makes the mustard yellow walls look a shade darker than they are. Our frugal habit of turning out all but every third ceiling light after 7:00 P.M. does nothing to enhance the emergency waiting area. A flower print with a frame but no glass hangs at a slight angle on the wall at one end of the room, lost in the wide expanse of dark yellow. In the corner a table holds magazines, dog-eared from last year. There appears to be no way to turn off the small color television suspended high on the wall out of reach.

"You got somebody sick?" asks the heavy blond woman with pale blue eyes and pink-white skin sitting next to me, holding a child in her lap, a big child of about nine, all gangling legs and arms lying against her mother in a spread of fatigue, her face buried in her mother's neck.

Her question startles me. Upstairs every bed has a patient in it. Carrie Williams was admitted yesterday for rapid heartbeat and shortness of breath. Coleman Forbes's sister slipped on a throw rug on her own back porch and knocked her head against the hot-water heater and lay unconscious on the floor for several hours with her arm broken until Coleman found her and called the ambulance. My neighbor Marcy Plummer brought her little boy into the emergency room last night. The child had a violent asthma attack and scared Marcy so badly she became hysterical and hurled herself against the glass-front cabinet in room 1, broke the glass, threw all the instruments on the floor, pulled open the drawers and emptied them in a heap, and then went after the IV cabinet before Charlene restrained her and guided her to the desk telephone at the back of the treatment room and told her to call and talk to as many people as she could think of, anywhere in the country, in the world even, free, while they took care of her child.

"No," I say. The woman means, Is somebody sick in my family? The hospital is not a family. "I work here. Thought I would sit a minute. What about you?"

"My husband's back there with bad chest pain. We're from Ohio. I wish we were home." The child raises her head briefly and gives me an expressionless look.

"There's a good doctor on tonight. Dr. Anderson. He is an internist with a subspecialty in emergency medicine, knows what he's doing. He will do everything possible for your husband. And a really good nurse. Her name is Charlene, and she has been an emergency room nurse for twenty years. You'll see her in a few minutes, a tall woman with dark curly hair wearing white slacks and a blue shirt. She's not dressed the way you might think a nurse should dress, but she is terrific."

What am I doing? Apologizing? The way I phrased it, she could interpret what I said to mean that there *happens to be* a good doctor and good nurse on tonight, that she is lucky, some other night there might be somebody "on" who does not know what he or she is doing.

Do I give her confidence in us by what I say? There is no way for me to know.

If you came this way to a strange town and saw a hospital with its lights on and doors open, would it mean to you that the hospital is good because if it were not, the town would have closed it down long ago? Can we count on the town to do that? On the state to withdraw a license from a hospital offering less than good care? On the Joint Commission to refuse to accredit or Medicare to refuse to certify? How does the public know? Only the presence or absence of a framed piece of paper hanging on the wall somewhere in the lobby—you could easily miss it on your way to the emergency room—stating that the hospital is accredited by the Joint Commission, which means that it is *far enough along in the process of* meeting a set of standards. How far along? And from which standards is the hospital still some distance? The piece of paper does not tell you that.

I could explain to this woman that we screen the credentials of all doctors on the medical staff. I could explain to her that no matter who is on duty we can always get hold of good doctors because they all live close by; we are small and in touch with them all the time. But that would imply that there are varied levels of competence among our doctors. The woman would listen but hear none of this, nor would it comfort her if she did hear—probably the opposite. She has one interest: a good outcome for her husband.

"What is your name?" I ask.

"Sharon," she says. "And this is Melinda." The child does not move. "My husband is Bud. Bud Grosholtz."

"Come up to my office and wait there, Sharon. We will get a cot for Melinda so she can lie down."

"No, I don't want to leave," she says.

"It's just upstairs. The nurse will call you."

"I can't leave."

We sit together in the semidarkness, and I look around the waiting area, my eyes getting used to the dim light. I could get up and turn on the remaining corridor lights, but then Sharon would have less privacy. The television—*Wheel of Fortune* relentlessly spinning high on the wall, there's Vanna White smiling—draws the eyes of the others away from Sharon. Noise and dinginess have their uses. On the other side of me is a middle-aged man, tan from the sun, wearing the summer colony uniform of oxford cloth shirt and madras shorts, his foot wrapped in a bandage. "Stepped on a damn rosebush," he says. "Thorn went right up into my foot. Hope there's somebody here who can get it out, and soon." Across the corridor two small boys wrestle giggling on the floor and pull on the trousers of a large man dressed in army fatigues with a wide canvas belt strapped around his middle and a dark beard covering most of his face. Next to him is his wife, Shirley, who works as a waitress at Rick's. I catch her eye. "He got bit," she says, pointing toward her husband. "An hour ago, in the woods. A raccoon bit him." Rabies, I am thinking, rabies is possible. I look anxiously back at the door to the treatment rooms, to see if someone is coming to get this man. No one is.

Next to Shirley, on an upright chair with a hard back, sits Tim Bailey. Is it a heart pain tonight, Tim? The summer evening is beautiful, the weather fine; then you must be quite ill. I wish Charlene would come.

Huddled together on another of our coffee-colored vinyl sofas sits a whole family, three adults and five children who look very much alike—large brown eyes, wary faces—watching and saying nothing. Who is hurt? I wonder. How far are they from home? Near them is Fred Ames, who works for the town plowing snow from the streets in winter and cutting back the long grass from the edge of the roads in summer. Next to him, Elizabeth Littlejohn, thin to extreme, dark circles under her eyes, admitted to the hospital six times in the last three months, with no insurance, but that is not the point; the point is that she does not improve. Next to her, Eddie Barnstone. Eddie is Bev Tracey's husband. He is a veteran of the war in Vietnam. Oh, Eddie, I hope you are not seriously ill, your wife is the best nurse we have, please stay well, Eddie, for yourself, my thoughts are first for you, do not get me wrong, but also for us so that Bev can work her regular shift, it is hard to find nurses as good as your wife. Next to Eddie, Mrs. Culbertson. Skip Culbertson's mother. A kind lady, so dignified, too old and frail to be sitting here. Why is she alone? Why isn't Art Seiler at this very moment making a house call to her summer cottage on the cliff above the rocks at the north end of the beach?

They all are having to wait more than an hour. That is too long. Why aren't we moving faster? Will every single one of them file suit against the hospital for nonattention and negligence? Or will they all die here, waiting, still waiting as they draw their last breaths?

We will hire another full-time emergency room doctor for the summer months. And two more nurses. Never mind cost containment; this long wait is an outrage.

We lost $90,000 on the emergency room alone last year. On the other hand, more than one third of admissions to the hospital come through the emergency room. Laboratory tests, X rays, electrocardiograms—our doctors order these in abundance for emergency patients. In abundance, I say. Do our doctors practice defensive medicine by ordering more tests than they actually need to diagnose the patient's condition? Yes, they do. An unknown patient is an unknown. An underlying condition conceals itself. If the doctor fails to discover it, he is considered negligent. To assure that no condition goes undiscovered, doctors order tests in abundance on emergency room patients whom they have never seen before. They can be more parsimonious with their own patients. With their own patients they already know a few things.

Charlene comes for Shirley's husband, and for Elizabeth Littlejohn, who walks mechanically behind her like a robot following an unchangeable program.

Father O'Malley appears suddenly, stops and looks at me, then turns slowly around and looks at the people waiting, then back to me and spreads his arms wide as if to offer a benediction. Please do, Father, I am thinking. Stand in this waiting room and pray for all those who are traveling, by land or sea, and for those who stay at home, and for all who wait for long hours in the emergency rooms of unknown small hospitals not knowing who will care for them when they are called.

"Why don't you put in a bar down here?" he shouts at me. "The best pub in town, here in the corner." This brings a big laugh from Eddie Barnstone, and once Eddie laughs and breaks the gloom the others begin to laugh also, all except Tim Bailey, who looks straight ahead, his legs crossed, his head cocked slightly to the side. I introduce Father O'Malley to the silent huddled family (they come from a town called La Pocatière on the shore of the St. Lawrence River), and then, after he has shaken hands and spoken to them all, and after they have told him that back in Canada they wouldn't have to pay—the government covers everyone and it's a lot cheaper and they are waiting just as long here as they would have to wait in Canada—I take his arm and steer him toward the treatment rooms, where we look for Bud Grosholtz.

The double doors at the end of the corridor swing open with a sudden clatter and a rush of people around a stretcher, some pushing the stretcher, some holding it back, this way, no, that way—"Over *here,* damn you," one familiar voice shouting above the others—too many people, too much shouting, the IV dangling wildly from its hook on the metal pole, Jim Boze leaning hard on his two hands to press down on the large form on the moving stretcher, resuscitating as he moves in sidestep alongside, breathing into the mouth of the form, then leaning hard again on the chest in steady rhythm. Art Seiler is pushing the end of the stretcher. "Out! *Get out!*" he shouts at us. "Wouldn't you know, a priest and an administrator, the last two creatures on earth—*move this patient, Move her!*" shouting at Dr. Anderson to pull Elizabeth Littlejohn's stretcher out of the cubicle in room 1 and move Big Scotty Milliken in, Seiler starting to intubate and Charlene's voice on the intercom to respiratory therapy, calling for blood gases, to the nursing floor for heated blankets. "In the river for twenty minutes, near drowning, skin pale, cold, patient not responsive. . . ."

"*Will* you move, please? Are you a nurse or some flower child?"

Dr. Anderson comes over to look at Scotty. "You'll want a heated blanket, warm oxygen depending on the blood gases, keep the IV going—I'd use Ringer's lactate. You might consider a steroid, single dose of methylprednisolone up to 500 milligrams, although there are no good data on it."

Dr. Seiler does a tap dance in the middle of room 1—quite good, graceful—then turns to face Dr. Anderson and bows deeply from the waist, sweeping his right arm all the way around from back to front in exaggerated motion as if it held a wide-brimmed hat with a feather.

"*Thank* you, Dr. Anderson."

Then he shoves his face into Dr. Anderson's. "You want to take care of this patient? What's the matter, you don't have enough income this month? Want me to give you a few more of my patients? Here, take them *all....*" He starts to push Scotty's stretcher away from the wall toward Dr. Anderson. Charlene grabs the stretcher with one hand and with the other holds tight to the oxygen tube connected from the wall to Scotty.

Dr. Anderson's flat expression does not change, but then it rarely does.

Big Scotty lies like a white whale on the stretcher.

I stop Jim Boze near the door. "What happened, Jim?"

"Would never happen in a million years, an old hand like Scotty, who's been lobstering all his life. Must have been tired, not watching himself. He brought his boat in later than usual and was standing on the town dock holding a line to the boat when he slipped off the edge. Apparently—Donny Whitworth and his cousin saw it, I didn't—Scotty grabbed the boat and hung on and the current pushed the boat suddenly and hard so that his legs were crushed between the boat and the edge of the dock. Then he fell in, and the current carried him fast upriver. In the water he could have grabbed hold of several mooring ropes, but he didn't even reach for them. He seemed to be unconscious, maybe from the pain in his legs, and at one point the current knocked him into one of the pilings of the bridge and kept him there straddling it long enough for Donny and his cousin to get to him and haul him into the skiff. Donny saw Dr. Seiler coming back down the river in his boat and hailed him, and they shouted at the truck driver on the dock to drive to the marina and call the ambulance. So that's two in one day."

"Two?"

"Yes. Scotty pulled Dr. Seiler out of the drink an hour before."

The curtains are pulled around Scotty. Connie from the lab pushes the curtain aside and hurries out with her metal basket of vials and needles. She looks at me but gives no signal, one way or the other.

"Will he make it?" I ask Jim.

"Might."

Bud Grosholtz lies on the second stretcher in room 1. When

he sees a priest coming toward him, he sits straight up and shouts for his wife to come and take him out of here; he has no intention of dying, and even if he does, he wants no priest praying over him. Father O'Malley tells him to shut up and lie down; he has no intention of praying anywhere near him. Father O'Malley walks past Bud and across the hall to room 2, where he pulls up a chair to sit with the family from La Pocatière, who are standing, all of them, stiffly and silently on either side of the next-to-youngest girl lying on the stretcher. In the next cubicle Charlene gives Shirley's husband shots for rabies, the big kind of shots requiring a long needle to the stomach muscles. Tim Bailey sits on a chair behind the curtain.

"There's a storm coming," Charlene says to me as she passes through the hallway.

"Really? Nothing on the TV news."

"It's coming. Tim Bailey is here. Weather will be only a few hours behind him."

"How does he know?"

"He always knows."

"You mean he's not sick? He just wants shelter?"

"He wants shelter all right. But his symptoms are real. Tim never fakes symptoms."

The radio in room 1 picks up a voice through distant static: "Male, about nineteen, motorcycle accident, multiple trauma, possible spinal cord injury, fifteen minutes, on our way."

Dr. Anderson stands by Bud's stretcher, expressionless.

"We want to keep you here for observation, Mr. Grosholtz. You have had a minor heart attack; you may have another; we will watch you carefully. Put you in a room upstairs with a monitor, to show the activity of your heart. Only a few days."

"There are no beds upstairs," Charlene says. "We'll have to keep him down here for a while longer."

"Sorry, can't stay, have to go," says Bud, swinging his legs over the side to stand up.

Dr. Anderson puts his hand on Bud's shoulder.

"Too great a risk for you to leave now," he says. "We'll make you comfortable as soon as we can. Let me speak to your wife."

"You leave my wife alone," Bud says. "I'll decide where I

stay and where I don't stay and I'm not staying here in this way station by the side of the road where nobody knows what they're doing, you and your dancing doctor friend arguing over a patient. What are you, some carnival band? You call this a hospital?"

Bud Grosholtz shoves Dr. Anderson away and stands up, puts on his trousers, his shoes without socks, and gathers up the rest of his clothes in a loose bundle. Still wearing his open-backed hospital gown, he walks past the nurse station and out into the waiting area corridor to Sharon. "Let's go," he says, and grabs her arm, and she grabs hold of Melinda as Bud pulls them along toward the door to the parking lot.

Charlene runs after them holding a clipboard. "Mr. Grosholtz, you are taking a very great risk, please think again. . . . Mrs. Grosholtz, can you persuade him?"

But Sharon is pulled forward on one side by Bud and on the other pulled back by a sobbing Melinda. Sharon takes hold of Bud's arm with both hands, digs her toes into the gravel of the parking lot, and with all her strength tries to stop him. Bud will not be stopped. Charlene tries to stand between Bud and the car door.

"At least will you sign this piece of paper, Mr. Grosholtz, which states that you are leaving the hospital *against medical advice*?"

Bud opens the car door against Charlene as if she did not exist and sits in the driver's seat. He starts the engine and backs out of the space, not even waiting for Sharon and Melinda, who climb into the back and are still closing the door as the car screeches forward.

I watch Charlene walk quickly back to the emergency room door. The ambulance pulls in just in front of her, and she helps Jim Boze open the back doors and ease out the stretcher holding the young motorcycle accident victim.

"About five miles north . . . double trailer truck swerved into the left lane and slammed him into the center railing . . . he went into a spin and was thrown double loop over the highway and into the ditch . . . truck bounced off the rail and into the right lane in front of a car . . . car forced into the ditch and ran over the boy . . . multiple body trauma, maybe spinal cord. . . ."

They wheel him into room 1, to the cubicle Bud has just vacated. All stations in all three rooms are occupied with patients. Dr. Anderson asks the man in the madras shorts with the thorn in his foot, who has hopped on one leg back to the door of room 1 of his own accord, to wait on a chair in the hallway. He will get to him as soon as he can. The man hops to the chair and stretches his suntanned leg out in front of him. Dr. Seiler leaves Big Scotty—breathing normally now, dry under his warm blanket—and comes over to look at the boy. Dr. Anderson has the intubation tube in place and heavy sandbags on each side of the boy's head to keep him still.

"Want me to take a couple of these other patients?" Seiler asks.

"No, thanks," Dr. Anderson replies.

"I advise you to transfer him right away," Seiler says. "Send him to Portland. Trauma unit—Dr. Salz—"

"You *what?*" says Dr. Anderson, leaning forward slightly as if he can't quite hear.

"I said I advise you to stabilize him and send him on. We can't handle it. We are not a trauma center."

"Well, thank you, Art, for your advice, but now that I'm here we just might become one," says Dr. Anderson.

Art Seiler begins to laugh. At first he laughs quietly, mouth closed, shoulders shaking slightly, his gleaming eyes fixed on Dr. Anderson. Slowly the laugh takes him over. His chest and belly jump, his mouth opens wide, and out comes a bellowing musical sound full of mirth and despair, cheer and exhaustion, every kind of emotion that accumulates in thirty years of summer and winter days and nights in this emergency room. Outside, the wind picks up suddenly and the sky darkens. Eddie Barnstone calls in a loud voice from room 3 to ask if anyone is coming to take care of him. He says he will kill himself here, instead of elsewhere, if no one comes immediately, and how would we like *that?* Would we like *blood on our hands?* That makes Art Seiler laugh even harder, and he goes into room 3 to sit down with Eddie. "Do you know what a trauma center is, Eddie?" he asks him, still laughing. "Let me tell you." Without waiting for an answer, he tells Eddie what a hospital has to have in order to be a trauma center, such accoutrements as a neurosurgeon—unless, of course, Dr. Anderson is already trained as a neurosurgeon and planning to expand his practice—and a bunch of special equipment, very expensive, Eddie, it would boggle your mind. . . . Eddie grabs Art Seiler by the neck and holds him in a stranglehold, at the same time shaking him as if he were to quiet him forever until Charlene and Jim Boze and Father O'Malley come running and pull them apart and ease Eddie into a chair. "So it's me you want to kill, not yourself, is that it?" Seiler says to Eddie, who stands up, picks up the chair he has been sitting on, and throws it out into the hallway and then slumps on the floor in the corner with his head against the wall, whimpering like a hurt animal.

The double doors swing open, and Sharon and Bud Grosholtz walk in with Melinda close behind, all drenched and soaked from the sudden heavy rain. Bud would see the chair flying out of the door of room 3 and crashing into the hallway except that his head is down and his eyes closed against the pain. "Bad pain again, in his chest and arm . . ." and Charlene and Dr. Anderson lift him onto a stretcher. "Put him in the ICU, I don't care who you have to move out, move him in, I'll get Dr. Burt to take him—"

"What! Giving away a patient?" Seiler says to Dr. Anderson, who ignores him.

The man with the rose thorn in his foot hops over to pick up the chair which has flown out of room 3 and landed in the hallway. He pulls it along to where he has been sitting and places it so that he can sit on one chair and prop his wounded foot on the other.

Jim Boze and Charlene wheel a stretcher holding the young motorcycle accident victim out the doors and quickly into the waiting ambulance, for the trip to Portland. The storm will slow them down, I think. Perhaps it will not last.

Dr. Sidney James walks down the corridor and into room 2 to the side of the young girl from La Pocatière surrounded by her silent family. He will take her to surgery right away to remove her appendix—that is, if her parents will sign a consent to surgery on her behalf. On a printed form attached to the clipboard, in the center of the page where there is a large white space, he draws the stick outlines of a human form and marks the spot, on the lower right abdomen, where he will cut into their daughter, a very small cut. They gather around him in a circle and stare at the drawing. He explains in a deliberate monotone voice the details and the risks of surgery, then holds out the clipboard and the pen. No one moves. None of the adults in the tight little group moves forward to sign. All stand silently, their eyes wide and scared. "We are wasting time," says Dr. James with patience. "I will explain again. . . ." Charlene calls Father O'Malley, who is sitting on the floor next to Eddie Barnstone. Father O'Malley hauls himself up slowly off the floor and comes next door.

"He's the best there is," Father O'Malley says to the family, gesturing his elbow at Dr. James. "Don't know quite what he's doing here, top academic surgeon, nothing he can't do, years of experience, good results. Go ahead and sign, you're lucky, better off than in Quebec I would think or anywhere else. Amazing that he's here . . ."

The eyes of the man with the thorn in his foot follow Dr. James as he wheels the young girl, her family holding tight on either side of the stretcher, down the corridor and out of sight.

Charlene brings Mrs. Culbertson into room 2. "Oh, my dear, you are so busy, I hate to bother you, but I felt faint and had some trouble catching my breath. . . . Oh, is that Dr. Seiler, is he here? . . . Dr. Seiler, I couldn't reach you, you must have been out on your boat, so I came to the emergency room. . . ."

"Ah, Mrs. Culbertson, are you here hoping to find me or do you want to see our new young Dr. Anderson the Neurosurgeon?"

"I didn't know. . . . Now that you're here, *can* you see me? . . . Oh, dear, have I done something wrong? . . . You must be terribly busy."

"Not too busy to see you, ever. Now, tell me what happened. . . ."

Dr. Anderson calls the nursing supervisor to find a bed for Elizabeth Littlejohn, who should be admitted immediately. He listens to some argument or discussion coming from the nursing supervisor Jessie Pace, and at one point he holds the telephone out and away from his ear and points to it so that we can hear Jessie's voice talking on and on to the air. At that moment lightning and a thunderclap on top of it strike with a deafening crack, and I wonder if Jessie can tell that the phone is not at Dr. Anderson's ear but held out for display and ridicule in the middle of room 1.

"Just find her a bed," Dr. Anderson is saying. "Move somebody. I don't care what you do; that's your problem. She is nauseated, excessively weak, signs of depression, electrolytes abnormal, don't like the look of her EKG, I intend to admit her."

"Grandfather threw her out of the house again, did he?" says Seiler, pointing toward Elizabeth as he comes into room 1 to Scotty, who is awake and showing some color in his face. "Need to get an X ray of your legs, Scotty, won't take long . . ." and Seiler starts to push Scotty's stretcher himself down the hall. He stops at room 3.

"Eddie Barnstone, give me a hand with Big Scotty. You're a strong fellow, help me get him to X ray. That emaciated little technician in radiology can't handle Scotty alone."

Charlene rushes up to Dr. Seiler. "Eddie Barnstone is a *patient*, presenting for *treatment*," she whispers, pulling Dr. Seiler away from room 3 so Eddie cannot hear. "Please leave him here. He is suicidal, and we have called for a psych consult; we must keep him under observation."

"Hasn't done it yet, has he?" Seiler shouts. "Hey, Eddie, you haven't killed yourself yet, have you?"

Eddie stops crying and stares at Dr. Seiler and, when Seiler moves on, stares at the wall, then slowly stands up and walks down the corridor toward X ray.

Dr. Anderson brings the man with the thorn in his foot into room 1 and closes the cubicle curtain. "Should I see a surgeon?" he asks. "Nah, we can get this," Dr. Anderson says. The radio broadcasts a distant voice: "Three-car accident, about fourteen miles south of you, bringing in two white females, one about . . ." The connection breaks. Only static. Then it comes back. ". . . with crushed pelvis, vital signs . . ."

Dr. Anderson goes over to the radio to broadcast instructions to the ambulance crew.

The double doors open and Coleman Forbes walks in, drenched from the rain.

"Coleman, I hope you are not here as a patient."

"Nope, just heard Art Seiler fell out of his boat and Big Scotty fell in the river and near drowned. Came to see how everyone is doing."

Tony comes up behind me.

"How's Scotty?"

"I think he's going to be all right," I say, and out of the corner of my eye I see Jack Mathias coming down the corridor from the other direction. Fred Ames, who cuts the long grass at the edge of the town roads in summer, comes out of room 2 with his arm bandaged to the shoulder, embarrassed to see this gathering of elite townsmen. "You okay, Fred?" asks Jack.

"Yes, just poison ivy," Fred says, looking sheepish and moving along quickly.

Through the double doors comes Skip Culbertson. His mother has been admitted.

"What's happening? Did Scotty make it?"

"Seems that way."

"They tell me we've got a fantastic new doctor in here."

"Actually, Art Seiler took care of him," says Coleman.

"Did you hear that?"

"Didn't have to hear it, I know it."

The four go to the meeting room to dry off. There might be some coffee left. I walk with them through the waiting area where the high-wall television blares sounds and images without interruption. All the seats are taken. A new group of patients has replaced the earlier one. Tony talks about marketing the emergency room.

"It's a center. Feature it. Make it a flagship," he says.

Jack says it's a loser and we can't throw money at a loser.

Skip says it's a necessity for those who live here and for those who winter over, and we should balance its losses with what it gains for us.

Coleman says: "Forget trying to balance everything, a bit here to this doctor for his favorite equipment, a bit to that one for political peace and quiet. Why not do something well? Take the long view."

"We always take the long view," says Jack.

I say good night and walk back through the waiting area. Sharon and Melinda are sitting on the vinyl sofa. I ask the nursing supervisor to put cots in my office for Bud Grosholtz's wife and daughter. Tomorrow we will find them a room in town. I see that Tim Bailey is lying on a stretcher in room 3. "We don't have a bed for him. He'll have to spend the night in here," Charlene says. In the hallway I pass Jack and Tony and Coleman gathering in front of the double doors.

"Where did this storm come from? There was nothing on the news," says Jack.

"Came out of the east, over the ocean, no warning," says Tony.

"Came out of nowhere," says Coleman.

EIGHT

Dear Tony,

Just a note to let you know we have started proceedings to evaluate the ability of Dr. Talley to practice in this hospital. He is behaving in a bizarre manner because of an alleged dependence on certain kinds of drugs. The medical staff has set up an ad hoc committee to investigate.

Tony, I hesitate to intrude on your retirement. Florida must be delightful—November is cold here, do I have to tell you?—and no one deserves a rest as much as you do. But I thought you would want to know this because you brought Dr. Talley and his partner, Dr. Burt, to the hospital in 1974, and these men are your good friends, your having gone through grim years together when you didn't know from one day to the next how long the doors of the hospital could stay open. From what others have told me, it was you who gave Dr. Talley a second chance, and out of gratitude to you he kept the hospital open.

We must take care of this doctor and get him to treatment. This is the reason for my letter.

Can you shed some light on those early years? I am told that within a month of the day Dr. Talley set up practice here there was a line of patients a mile long in front of his office door, waiting to see the brilliant new internist who diagnosed conditions left (as he said) for years untreated. He has an even larger following of devoted patients now. Donny Whitworth stopped me in the drugstore yesterday and talked for twenty minutes about the miraculous Dr. Talley and how he is a new man since Dr. Talley "agreed to take him as a patient." Agreed to take him! Can you believe that? Every one of our doctors is looking for patients to fill the narrow-lined spaces on their schedule books, and Dr. Talley, even with his following, is no exception. Donny, however, believes he is in the company of the chosen. His loyalty is strong—typical of Dr. Talley's patients. Over at Rick's, at breakfast and almost anytime, you can see him talking with a group of friends, and I will wager that he is talking about Dr. T. and the hospital, there being nothing very urgent in town to talk about at the moment other than the charter and the growth ordinance. We need you back to stir up some excitement.

It is late to be dictating a letter, nine-thirty on a Friday evening. Even Gerry has reluctantly gone home. Before leaving, she leaned through the office door and advised me to seek balance in my life. But this is the time to find some order in words. In the blessed quiet of the hospital night there is little disturbance. Bev is on tonight, finishing the end of a double shift. Dr. Talley stopped at the mailbox wall an hour ago.

It is more than loyalty with his patients. More like a hypnotized band of cult worshipers, who, though they are not all friends of one another, could in an instant bind themselves together with hoops of steel against any action to reduce Dr. T.'s privileges in the hospital or remove him from the medical staff, and do not think they won't know about it ten minutes after it happens.

But we can't afford him. The risk for *potential* harm is more than we can carry. The man is too volatile. He is a tray slammer, like certain medical center doctors—exhausted, controlled, stone-faced—who wait silently in the cafeteria line until they reach the stack of wet plastic trays, grab a tray, and slam!—the cracking sound of plastic tray hitting the hollow steel pipes of the tray line counter echoes down the lunch line.

We have the same wet plastic trays and tubular steel in our cafeteria, but here the counter is short, and the frail elderly volunteer who receives our money at the end of the lunch line is too close. The slam frightens her, blasts her eardrums. We can't afford tray slammers here.

Tony, as you know, the hospital has a legal obligation to protect patients from *predictable* harm. Dr. Talley has made no serious mistakes, but the potential is there. The rumor is that he takes both uppers and downers. His behavior lacks balance. On some days he walks a straight line with a serious look. But it doesn't last. The next day he is on a high, behaving erratically. He staggers slightly, and his hands shake. Laughs uncontrollably when there is nothing funny. One morning last week he came to the emergency room looking as if he had spent a week under the table in a whorehouse kitchen. Then there are brief moments of rage, one yesterday in the cafeteria tray line over nothing, nothing at all. He has lost a lot of weight since you last saw him.

This is a problem to be handled carefully. I must be patient, cut the risk and find a solution but not too fast. The medical staff is reluctant to take action against a colleague, although physicians are required by law to report unusual behavior to the state licensing board. The snitch law, they call it. I am pushing them to do so and am accused daily of vindictiveness and meddling. One reason they hesitate, I believe, is an important one. Dr. Talley is a genius at diagnosis, and every one of his colleagues here knows it and asks his advice. Without him several would be up a creek. The end result of his care of patients is high on the scale according to the explicit clinical criteria of our new quality assurance program. If he leaves, the level of quality in this hospital, on paper and in fact, will go down.

In Tony's years as chief executive of a large urban medical center, he must have watched doctors like him, many of them, fold up under the stress of medical practice. Of the physicians who enter treatment programs, the highest number are internists, the specialty that faces daily the most painful illnesses.

But (studies show) far more significant than the ills of their patients are factors of childhood and personal stress. What can I know about a doctor's deprived childhood from an interview? Ask about it? Absurd. But it comes down to a need for information before we encourage or discourage a doctor to apply for privileges here. We are a small hospital, vulnerable to the whims and behavior of individuals.

All we know is what is on a doctor's record and what we learn from phone calls to his or her former hospitals and to state licensing boards.

Tony, if he asks you to find him a place in another state to which he can flee, where he can obtain a license and hospital privileges in some small hospital like this one where the administrator is desperate for a physician, please do not set it up for him. He needs immediate treatment. Both James and Seiler will talk to him tomorrow. If he calls you (he may have already), would you throw your weight toward his going into one of the impaired physician treatment programs, any of them? Georgia has a good one, and so does Oregon. I am very concerned. He looks like a potential suicide.

Just out of curiosity, where did you find these two doctors? (I will change their names in this letter in case Dr. T. decides to sue the hospital for removing his means of livelihood.) Are they beholden to you? You never did tell me the whole story.

Talk about risk!

Some impaired physicians gravitate to small hospitals, where they think they will be so badly needed that the hospital credentials committee will relax its standards. But with Tony here that could not have happened. There was, I know from the record, an organized medical staff in place shortly after Tony came in 1972. Dr. Seiler was president, and then there was a Cuban surgeon, who has since vanished. They must have reviewed the credentials of these two and voted favorably. Tony must have told Seiler that Drs. T. and B. were first-class physicians who simply needed a second chance. And he was right. I know that.

Tony told me that a few weeks after he moved here to retire, he was working quietly in his garden when Jack Mathias
drove up to his house and asked him to come in and manage
the hospital. The board had no one for the job, the last fellow,
called The Clerk, having left without notice. There were four
patients in the hospital, three lawsuits pending (two against the
Cuban surgeon), and insufficient funds for the payroll. Tony
said it looked like fun. He accepted immediately. But he had
been forty-some years in this business. Wasn't he ready for a
rest? And what's so much fun about it?

Tony must have known a lot about the quality of their medical practice to get these two past Seiler, quality that did not
show in their dismal record of hospital privileges lost, licenses
suspended, bankruptcy, divorce, child support suits. The risk
was too great otherwise. But the risk of doing nothing was
even greater. Not to bring doctors here, the kinds of doctors
who would immediately attract patients to the hospital, would
have meant closing the doors. If Tony had gone about it the
usual way—a recruitment committee, Seiler in charge, numbers
on a newsprint flip chart about physician-population ratios
and negative growth and how they were losing "market
share"—then he could have reasoned with Seiler. Reasoned
and gotten nowhere. There wasn't time; it would have taken
months. The hospital would have closed before the committee
had gotten around to its first meeting. He did it the only way
possible: just moved the two of them in, smiling his enigmatic
smile and talking in grand terms (but credible, nobody speaks
with more credibility than Tony) about forming a multi-
specialty group practice that would bring in more income for
Dr. Seiler and the Cuban surgeon than they in their solo practices had ever dreamed of. Seiler would thrive on the intellectual stimulation of having two bright internists on the staff. He
could lunch with them daily and discuss the latest medical research findings.

The two knew how to admit patients to the hospital. There
is nothing they didn't know about wording a medical record in
the language of "appropriate utilization of inpatient hospital
services" to convince Medicare and Blue Cross to pay the bill.
A patient could go to one of them with a cut finger and find

himself in room 23 for a four-day stay. Hospital admissions increased by 400 percent in the first three months after their arrival. There were patients in beds in the corridors. "Never turn a patient away," Tony said once. "Find a place for him somewhere. Put him in the phone booth if you have to." Drs. B. and T. took over the emergency room and admitted everyone who walked in the door. The board loved the new cash flowing into the hospital. The hospital licensing board approved Tony's proposal to convert some long-term care beds in the Shipley Wing to acute care. Tony could sell sand to a beachcomber.

Then, after a year, when the hospital was thriving, Tony reined in his high-stepping ponies and told them to slow down and behave like normal physicians. And they did just that. No one was hurt except the Medicare Trust Fund and a couple of insurance companies that paid the cost of unnecessary patient days. Tony explained to the board that the continuing survival of a small hospital meant *lower* costs to these insurers in the future because the very same patients who were here now would have gone instead, if we were not here, to one of the larger regional hospitals whose costs were at least 40 percent greater than ours. Actually, as his argument went, he did Medicare a favor.

What I admire about you, Tony, among many things, is the way you jump into a risk without hesitation, your lightning-swift mind having already weighed all the gains and losses in a single instant. You make your choice and run with it—one of your strokes I want to adopt for my own.

Hospitals used what they had, back in the glory days of the sixties and seventies, and Medicare cost reimbursement was what they had. We all were good at milking the most out of Medicare, clever at maximizing revenue. Why not? What reason did we have to be efficient? On the contrary, what we spent on whatever was reasonable (optimal) for patient care flowed right back to us. There were some good tricks in those days. To maximize reimbursement, we could manipulate the old Medicare cost-finding formula called Ratio of Charges to Charges Applied to Cost. Divide Medicare patient charges by total patient charges; that was one ratio. Multiply that by total "allowable" costs, and that gave us a cost figure to be reimbursed by Medicare. Well, we could (I won't say any of us *did*) mark up the charges in departments heavily used by the elderly, like the pharmacy, to get a higher numerator in that first figure and a higher total. And then there was the Exploding Price Code. The clinical laboratory used a code to represent a particular lab test and the price charged for it. A CBC (complete blood count) could be coded as one test with a charge of $17. But explode the price code into three separate components of the CBC: HP (hematology profile) without platelets, $9.30; platelet count, $6.20; differential, $5.60. Separately these added up to $21.10. The whole was less than the sum of its parts. Separate the parts, line them up to be counted, and Medicare would pay. There were all kinds of things like that.

We were so busy manipulating revenue we hardly had time to notice the basic services we were not providing.

But we played according to the rules Medicare set up for us. It was all for the patient's benefit. We strengthened the services Medicare would pay for, ignored the ones it would not. Take respiratory therapy, for instance. In the old days nurses performed respiratory treatment. Technicians called respiratory therapists were no more than a gleam in a pulmonary physician's eye, but Medicare paid the costs of their separately defined services, and miraculous! a whole new profession was born, complete with body of knowledge, certification, skill levels, and lists of equipment as long as your arm. The cost of nurses, however (except for a token differential), fell into a category called routine service, a lumpen mass of room and board and "routine" nursing on which Medicare set cost limits. Nurses were not featured under Medicare; they were buried. Salaries for nurses remained so low they could have been under the ground. Even so, hospital costs continued to rise.

Tony, I am curious about something. Back in the days of the open faucet of cost reimbursement, what kept the costs of *this* hospital from rocketing into the stratosphere? Could it have had something to do with an initial condition, a tendency toward frugality . . .

Tony came here just in time for the dismantling of price controls on health care. Richard Nixon imposed price controls under the Economic Stabilization Program in 1971 and revoked them in 1974. Tony got the brunt of the sudden increase in the cost of everything—wages, supplies, equipment— brought on by the lifting of price controls. Regulation failed to control the rising cost of medical care.

... or was your hand so fine that you knew exactly where to spend money and where not? You talked about a hospital without walls, started a home care agency, put money into weight loss and stop smoking classes, meals on wheels—unglamorous low-tech things aimed at long-term improvement in health. The people here enjoy the benefit of your forward thinking.

But Tony missed one trick: He didn't circle it fast enough. The game tripped up some of its best players, even Tony. He kept his costs low, and in 1978, when Jimmy Carter threatened to place a cap on hospital revenues, panic set in, and hospitals—on the advice of the Big Eight accounting firms, which said, "Get your cost base *up,* you wanna be capped at a *low rate?*"—dutifully inflated their budgets (in the name of adequate staffing, state-of-the-art equipment, and quality) and jacked up their costs as high as possible before the cap could lock them into a level of reimbursement lower than neighboring hospitals, all the while talking about a "voluntary effort" among hospitals to control costs. Tony may have been so far ahead of the game that he knew what would happen. The cap never came because the AMA opposed it, the voluntary effort was just that, voluntary, and hospital costs continued to rise.

Even when Ronald Reagan introduced market competition to the health field, regulation did not go away. Some of it shifted to the states. The work of the Maine Health Care Cost Review Board began as genteel budget review. Like Blue Cross, it was started by the hospitals themselves to show good faith in cost control and turned into a three-headed monster that regulates, by state statute, hospital spending based on its 1983 costs. Well, our costs weren't high *enough* in 1983! Now we

suffer, capped by the state at a low level. We weren't playing
the game.
The incentives of the market would control costs.

Tony, even before incentives became a factor, didn't you
almost succeed in starting a health maintenance organization here? You had it in place. But it was too soon. You
were too far ahead.

A health maintenance organization (HMO) is based on incentives in reverse of fee-for-service: Be efficient, keep patients
well, and reduce their need for expensive care. In an HMO a
group of physicians accepts responsibility for a group of patients who pay yearly premiums for a range of services. The
less spent on patients, the more money the group retains.
Tony would have succeeded except for two key factors.
Private-practice physicians boycotted HMOs from the beginning. To protect fee-for-service medicine, some physicians
would go to any lengths, including dusting off and trotting out,
one more time, the doctor-patient relationship. And secondly,
Tony's HMO offered too many expensive services to too few
patients at too much distance. Again, it came down to what it
always was, a matter of size and volume. We were just too
small.
Do we have a second chance? The intent of competition is
this: that health insurance plans will seek out the most efficient
doctors and hospitals, providing the highest-quality care at
lowest cost, and contract with them for care of their beneficiaries. The public will choose health plans based on quality and
cost. But what is quality in the mind of the public? A hospital
without the latest technology might be low in cost, but people
see it as low in quality. How do we send a message that our
quality is geared to basic care and judgment?
Another thing I admire about Tony is his sense that time
moves slowly here. While other hospitals rushed to "restruc-
ture" themselves, in the fashion of the late seventies, to spin off
for-profit subsidiaries like spokes of a spider's web shaking in
the wind, to enter businesses unrelated to health care—motels,
parking lots, consulting firms—full of the promise of revenue

(and little result), he and Jack Mathias and Art Seiler stayed with basic hospital care. And they were right. That whole movement was another false game. Hospitals have returned to simple governing structures designed for care of the sick and injured.

Back to Dr. Talley. Do not think for a moment I am unaware of the bind you were in back in 1974, when quality meant having the doors of the hospital open and the lights on. I can talk now about quality as the act of discouraging a questionable doctor from even considering setting up a practice in this town ("too full, overdoctored, you'll never make a living here"), but I was not here in those days and not in your shoes.

This matter is tragic because I have seen Dr. T. in the very act of medical practice, and I have never seen better. He can sense instantly what is wrong with a patient. There is a connection, a bond between them; he feels what the patient feels, I know it.

I have been watching Dr. Talley with patients in the emergency room. I watch him frequently. This afternoon he treated a patient in acute pulmonary distress, an elderly man thin to the bone with a pale, transparent face sunken into his skull except for a protruding beak nose. It was Joe Littlejohn, who sits all day on the bench by the lobster and fish house next to the town wharf. He was in a state of breathless terror, gasping and straining for air. Joe has a medical history as long as the chart itself: severe anemia, hypertension, an acute myocardial infarction eight months ago, arthritis in his upper extremities. Dr. T. had Joe sitting upright on the stretcher with legs dangling, and as he moved the stethoscope over Joe's back, he said something, and Joe laughed. It was impossible, a patient can't laugh if he can't breathe, but he did. Dr. T. moved fast and easily around the stretcher with no wasted motion, keeping one hand on the patient without tangling with the respiratory therapist, who had set up oxygen and was drawing blood, or with Joe's ten-year-old grandson, who was clinging with clenched white fingers to the edge of the stretcher. Joe kept his eyes on Dr. T.

as he moved, and Dr. T. kept his eyes on Joe, breaking contact only once to look down the room directly at me standing in what I thought was an inconspicuous corner and do a mock stagger dance for my benefit (he knew I was watching him), pretending to lose control by rolling his eyes up into his head and bending his knees as if he were going to fall (Joe laughed, again!), then after that never lost contact with his patient.

The man is good, Tony. He is connected; he concentrates. It is a shame, a waste of talent. I hope you agree to help us.

One problem for a medical center doctor who flees to a small hospital is the sudden slowdown. It is more than just culture shock. It is a shock to his system, a complete change of pace. The lack of stress itself is stressful, more serious than simple boredom. Dr. T. likes to be exhausted; he is at his best then. Here there are not enough patients to exhaust him. And there is another problem. Medical centers can and do surround and cover a doctor who is showing signs of impairment, at least for a while. We cannot do that here. Our doctors practice in a glass house where every move they make is known instantly by every single hospital employee, and in the next few minutes most of the people in town are discussing it.

If we could, we would keep Dr. T. here on salary as a pet diagnostician and limit his privileges to seeing patients only under the supervision of another physician. But the budget will not allow it.

Tony, nothing bad has happened. Dr. T. has made no gross errors that we know of. But if a disaster occurs in the care of a patient, the hospital is liable for not predicting, from the evidence at hand, that it would happen.

Through the open door I hear unusual sounds coming from the nurse station and run out to check. Bev is holding Dr. T. in her arms and trying to ease him into a chair. He weeps uncontrollably in long, high, wailing screams as if calling to someone far away who cannot hear him. Bev holds him, and I grab hold, too, but he slides past the chair and onto the floor under the nurse station counter, where he lies in a half-stretched half-fetal position. Bev telephones Dr. B. to come immediately. We sit on the floor with Dr. Talley, holding his hand, speaking in brief phrases, listening to his sobbing. Dr. B. persuades him to stand up. They walk outside.

"Miss Janssen is back," Bev tells me. "She did so well for a while. From her room on the ground floor at Gertrude McKinnon's house she could see the river and a bit of the ocean beyond the trees. Dr. Talley talked her into radiation therapy, drove her himself every week to Bangor. Then a sudden failing today . . . We've admitted her; she is in a lot of pain."

Miss Janssen's face is so pale the white pillowcase seems dark underneath it. A sharp cry from the woman in the next bed wrenches Miss Janssen hard, as if the pain had traveled like lightning across the divide between the two beds.

"I asked for a private room for her, but she heard me and said no, please, she wanted to stay in this room."

"I must listen to people in pain," Miss Janssen says. "Now that I have my own pain, you see, I have made a discovery. The pain I was imagining in others was not their whole pain but only a part of it. My imagination was not keen enough to know how bad it was, and so all those years I wasn't with my imaginary companions at all, I was still an outsider."

"For God's sake, Bev, can't she have a shot?"

"She refuses it. Ask Dr. Talley."

Miss Janssen continued. "And then I discovered something else. I was imagining pain to be worse than it was because I did not take into account the drowsiness and reverie, the way the mind travels, the qualifying circumstances. I have my own pain now and know better. The lady next to me is in terrible pain, but something mitigates it. I asked Dr. Talley if I had it right. 'Right, doctor?' I said."

Tony, have you always been able to hold on to your enthusiasm? Or have you lost it on occasion and retrieved (or regenerated) it by starting over a second or third or fourth time, when someone gave you, or you gave yourself, another chance? That is what you gave Dr. T. by bringing him up here, and it turned out almost all right. Almost. Will you give him a third (or is it a fourth) chance? But of a different kind this time? If he agrees to treatment, he can be spared adverse action by his colleagues. I will try to get him to the Georgia program which goes from a ninety-six-hour detox to a rehabilitation institute, a halfway house, then outpatient treatment. It lasts twenty months, and at the end the patient (doctor) is assigned to a mission where he treats patients with his own disease in "mirror image therapy." I have a notion that Dr. T. already sees himself mirrored in many of his patients.

The game has changed. The National Practitioner Data Bank, mandated by the Health Care Quality Improvement Act, holds information on any adverse action against licensed physicians (and other licensed health practitioners) reported to a state licensing board. So you see, all this jumping and fleeing and slipping out from under to a new untried area before their present colleagues take action is over for doctors like Dr. T. To help him now, we have to do it differently. The medical staff will offer him a hearing. If he does not appear, then the matter is closed. We notify the state licensing board.

As usual we need your help. You have a way with him. He'll listen to you.

His colleague Dr. B., you will be happy to know, has settled into a steady practice here. His patients swear by him. Did you know it would turn out this way? Treat him as if he were a first-rate doctor and he becomes one. (How often can we count on that?) He can make a living seeing ten or twelve patients in his office a day, plus a night a week on the emergency room and fees for reading EKGs. More than that would be too much for him; he is painfully shy. He doesn't "market" himself at all, but when it comes to knowledge, the other doctors seek him out. Lately they have started to go to him for consultation. Every evening he is here in the hospital library reading journals. Research is what he likes. In fact, I want to help him set up a small research lab here. Small hospitals should become part of the medical research network, don't you think? They are natural settings for studies over the long term, to determine what practice patterns affect outcome most positively. It would mean applying for a grant. Your ideas are more than welcome.

A doctor has to want to practice here for reasons other than those of a fugitive. He has to like elderly patients, not be bored by chronic illness, like to read. Are there such doctors? Yes, there are. We have several. A less than competent doctor lasts a short time here because his failings cannot be hidden. You could say this is one aspect of quality care at small hospitals. One of our strengths. At the same time an overly competent, high-achieving academic physician—I am thinking of Dr. James, who has done wonders for the reputation of this hospital—is in danger of stagnation and professional loneliness and a notion that he is slumming.

Our new doctors are suited to rural practice. They want to raise their children here and own a sailboat. Some spend a lot of time on their boats in summer, leaving Seiler to cover their practices and the emergency room, but that is not a problem. The other day Coleman asked me if I knew what a lifestyle is. I said no, I did not, and Coleman said he didn't either, but Dr. Anderson has a lifestyle. He is building a barn himself, has already drawn the plans and started digging the foundations with his hand shovel, has his two little boys out digging, too. Wants to get his friends together for a barn raising. He brings his newborn baby to medical staff meetings in a pouch hanging on the front of his chest. Relaxed, family-centered. It's like looking at the future and liking what you see.

Everything is changing, Tony. The old order is upside down. Are we off the mark when we define physician incentives as strictly financial? Money, science, lifestyle. How do we determine the right mix?

But you are ahead of me, as always, reading this long letter and laughing to yourself. What I most admire about you is your style—your grace—in paying court to the old kings, lavishing attention on physicians long after they have lost their political power (business, the payer, has it now, and perhaps the public), treating them with a kindness that gathers them in without their even knowing that specialization has separated them from their patients, that they are shells of what they could be with a wider vision, that greed and exhaustion and the unmitigated pain of others have driven them into the ground.

You think in terms of the whole. Somewhere in the past you picked up the old systems structure and carried it with a giant leap into the future, leaving behind the notion that every patient is reduced to a category, that the environment is a distant enemy firing at us. In the scientific theory called *chaos* (maybe you have left that behind, too, and are on to the next, *complexity*), the system and the environment are one and the same. That means that a frontier design, even a small one, could change both. For example, members of a cooperative like the local farmers' Grange were both consumers and providers. Or take the ideas of Paul Ellwood, the physician, and Alain Enthoven, the economist whose articles you used to copy for me from the *New England Journal of Medicine*. Throughout the decade of the seventies these two wrote about consumer and provider sharing the risk of illness, and about competition between "organized systems." How many decades will it take us to organize and deal with risk?

At least I can let these ideas ride at the back of my mind like weightless crystals. They can't do any harm, the way things are going. You always thought it important to keep the hospital open, and I agree.

Thanks, Tony, in advance, for your help with Dr. T. We must take care of our own doctors. They know a lot about medicine. I hope you are enjoying your new life in Florida.

It is Saturday morning and I am writing a second letter to Tony:

Dr. T. left yesterday without notifying his office or arranging for another doctor to cover his patients in the hospital. Miss Janssen died early this morning in great pain. Dr. T. left sixteen hospital medical charts incomplete with no progress notes, four of them lacking a dictated history and physical. We do not have a key to his office to get in and find records for patients to take to another doctor. A locksmith is coming to open the door, but it will be late this evening before he is able to do the job.

If Dr. T. contacts you, would you ask him to call and give me an address, or better yet a telephone number, where Dr. B. can reach him for consult on these patients whose treatment Dr. T. has started but the outlines of which are difficult to understand from his handwriting in the chart?

NINE

Monday morning, six-thirty. A dark April morning, the air heavy with snow. Last night's weather report said the storm was coming from the southeast. Its center would cross the coast a hundred miles south of here. We should expect six or eight inches of snow and a forty-mile-per-hour wind. Nothing to be concerned about.

But already there is a foot of snow on the ground and a lot more falling. I leave the car at home and walk to the hospital, a ten-minute walk on a good day but longer in weather. At the turn of the hospital driveway I see the headlights of the town snowplow coming toward me along the main street. I wave to the driver, Fred Ames, and signal him toward the hospital. But it is not Fred driving; it is the new town manager himself. His name is Hobart.

Hobart is king of the mountain high in the cab of the giant snowplow. He is from away, I do not know what place, but this morning he has the town to himself. As he moves under the streetlight, I can see his red and black plaid Maine hunting cap and pale, eager face through the clear glass triangle drawn by the windshield wiper. He opens the door of the cab, and even before I climb up, he begins the argument, the same argument we have had since he arrived in town three months ago.

"The town does not plow the hospital drive because the

hospital rests on seven acres of choice midtown property not on the tax rolls. Buy your own snowplow. Clear your own asphalt."

"Hobart, listen, half the homeless of the town and county are in the emergency room this very minute, even as we argue. I'll buy a plow when you build a shelter."

"If we plow you out this morning, I will have to charge you."

"Fine, and I will send the town a bill for service fees to the hospital as holding area, social service agency, food storage bank, fallout shelter, disaster planner, and largest employer in town, without which the economic health of this town would diminish, more than diminish, Hobart—*sink into the ground*."

"We will challenge the tax-exempt status of the hospital."

"Challenge it. We give away so much free care the courts will award us overflowing buckets of tax exemption just to keep us doing what we're doing."

"Maybe we can negotiate. . . ."

"Anytime."

Hobart turns and plows slowly toward the door, where I climb out and thank him many times. He will plow the driveway and the parking lots. With this much snow we will need him again later. He says he will come back.

Gerry is already here.

"Gerry, did you walk in?"

"I was here late and heard the last weather report, so I slept in the emergency room."

The ultimate devotion to duty. She wins.

"Look, we have trouble. Eddie Barnstone went to the floor to find Bev and announced he was ready to drive any nurse who needs a ride in this snow, his jeep is gassed up to go. He followed her in and out of patients' rooms, stomping his boots, the bulk of him dropping snow over charts and bedside tables, looming over their beds as the patients woke up, you know how he is, 'Let's get this show *moving*. Do I drive or do I not?'—you know he and Bev are separated and she wants a divorce—harassing her in front of patients until she gave him the names of three nurses who live miles away from each other, the other ends of the earth as far as driving in this snow."

"Maybe Eddie will bring one nurse in at a time instead of driving them all around to pick up the others."

"Do you think so?"

Gerry and I make rounds together, walking down the narrow stairway and left into the long corridor leading to the emergency room. Tiles missing from the corridor ceiling reveal a cat's cradle of pipes and wires and cables, tangles of lines of every material and diameter, every age and purpose, some of them leading in a sure direction and others with no fathomable intent whatsoever. Now that the hospital has three wings instead of two, there is no one best way to go from one place to another. To walk from the 1958 building to the new emergency room, Gerry and I can choose either the old corridor past the meeting room or the Caleb Wing connector. We can no longer see everyone on our way, as half go one way and half the other. For face-to-face exchange we substitute telephone messages, memos, notes left in mailboxes, scheduled appointments. Soon the computer system will have a "mailbox," messages to be retrieved by one's staring into a bottomless blue screen until the message appears. More efficient, Pete tells me, less cumbersome than all that immediate firsthand information.

We pass the door of central sterile supply and see Betty Janis, the new technician hired exclusively to keep track of Dr. James's surgical instruments, gowned and surrounded by blue linen as if underwater. She waves from her sterile world. In the corridor we meet Dr. James. He and the new operating room supervisor from Florida have been getting along splendidly. If you measure quality by order, efficiency, nurse satisfaction, rapid turnaround time, low rate of infection, minimal disturbance, as well as good results for patients, the quality of care in the operating room is high.

But lately, it seems, Dr. James moves in a world of his own, noticing others only at the periphery. At the same time he is more patient with us. He takes time to explain certain facts of medicine to me. Yesterday in the meeting room I showed him a list of equipment requested by the new cardiologist. A Holter monitor—for measuring and recording the activity of a patient's heart—costs $68,000 with computer. Does he need this?

"You see, the heart is a muscle. . . . It contracts in a certain way. . . . Heart activity is measured in sharp peaks and valleys recorded on a small device strapped around the patient's chest to keep a record of what he is doing every hour for twenty-four hours. The recording is then run through a computer in the hospital to match heartbeats to the patient's waking and sleeping, work and rest. It's a lovely device, pure quality."

"Yes, but does he *need* it?"

"Well now, think of it this way. He needs it about the way a carpenter needs a level."

"A level? But a carpenter *has* to have a *level*."

"Well, there you are."

His reputation is superb; his fame has spread. A hospital with Dr. James on its staff is a good hospital.

"Good morning, Dr. James. The snow is really coming down."

"Good morning. Yes, a lot of snow. Say, if you are going to be in your office later on, I will stop by. Something I must tell you. . . ."

Gerry and I turn right off the old corridor into the connector to the Caleb Wing. Suddenly everything is brighter, the walls and woodwork newly painted. The connector slopes downward to adjust for the difference in floor levels between the old and new buildings, giving us the intense pleasure of walking downhill, just for a minute. Through the large window on the south side I can see each snowflake outlined in the early half-light.

The Caleb Wing is seven months old, handsome and full of mistakes. Like so many chattering ghosts, the mistakes and shortcomings, things we left out (to reduce the cost), things we added (to suit one or another doctor whom we want to keep here forever), decisions and compromises follow us through the bright clean halls and rooms of the new building. Why isn't the treatment room closer to the nurse station? Gerry wants to know. Why do we need a second treatment room? It is a gift of convenience to the doctors who use it, free, to see their own private office patients, using the hospital's supplies, free, with free help from hospital nurses. Am I aware of this?

"Doctors are our customers."

"What are nurses? Your servants?"

"Slaves to quality."

Gerry stops in her tracks and unleashes a torrent of accumulated rage. For shelter, the triangular building offers us a sharply pointed corner waiting room narrower by degrees than a rectangle's corner. We stand eyeball to eyeball. Gerry demands two seats for nurses on the board of trustees—"long overdue and only logical since the reason a patient is *in* the hospital is for nursing care." I say for what I have in mind she should find at least six nurses of leadership quality to run for election to a new kind of governing body where information on health needs is considered, with much argument. Scour your crowd, I say, and find nurses who can make a case for programs to match the problems. Gerry says she doesn't have that kind of material on her staff because of the salaries we pay. Redefine material, I say. Gerry says no nurse at *this* hospital can grow professionally because of the excessive burden of nonnursing tasks that could easily be done by some lesser-trained person, freeing nurses to practice nursing. I say look at the mix of aides and licensed practical nurses on the staff. She says she would rather hire an R.N. any day. I walk ahead and Gerry stays with me like an angry demon, a dybbuk determined to enter my consciousness and fill it with a black foam of wrongs and injustices, mistakes, incompetence. Why doesn't the linen cart have its own alcove? The triangular shape of the building is disorienting. Didn't we anticipate that? We are accustomed to rectangles. Why is the nurse meeting room no more than a closet? What happened to the storage room for ventilators, the satellite pharmacy? ("Those were cut from the plans long ago." "Really? No one told *me*.") Why should doctors have six telephone dictating stations on the floor? So that doctors never have to wait? Customers must not be kept waiting.

Gerry and I are quiet as we approach the emergency room. We both have many new opportunities for error. Mistakes bury each other, fortunately.

Charlene is at the nurse station, talking on the phone.

". . . okay, so far, Jeanie, Eddie Barnstone is on his way to get you. . . . No, don't stand out on the road, not in this storm. . . . He knows where you live. Bev gave him directions. . . ."

Dr. Anderson looks up from the chart propped against his knees, which are bent to allow his feet to rest on top of the desk behind the counter and his chair to tip back almost to the point of lost balance and backward flip. Dr. Anderson has become a listener. In the last few months his manner has changed; he shows interest in what is said to him. More thoroughly concerned. (How studied is this change? I wonder. No, I am wrong, it is genuine.) He draws patients into his ever-burgeoning practice by listening. Six or eight empty styrofoam coffee cups litter the desk. Through the window behind his head I can see Hobart's snowplow as it clears the emergency room entrance, the heavy snowflakes covering the cleared road as fast as Hobart can plow it.

Tim Bailey is in the corridor. I ask Dr. Anderson to save beds, if possible, for storm victims. Tim could have a cot in the firehouse. Dr. Anderson says that Tim is sick, and Elizabeth Littlejohn needs a bed also. Also, a family came in an hour ago with a fifteen-year-old, looks like an appendix. Dr. James will do it in the next twenty minutes.

In the intensive care unit, Pauline Legere, Clinical Nurse Specialist, rests her head on the counter among a bank of monitors surrounding her like a black halo. Jagged lines of green lightning move across the screens left to right in steep or shallow peaks and valleys according to the heartbeat of the patient connected to the monitor by a tiny wire.

"Mrs. Culbertson went into cardiac arrest about one-thirty and Dr. Anderson called a full code and we got a tube and an IV line in her and a bag going while he shocked her back with the defibrillator, that delicate, dignified lady. . . . We pounded and pummeled her, and her heart came back—but the bruises, I can't bear the *bruises*—"

The fatigue of the last hours is all over her.

"—Mrs. Culbertson's family wants her to die peacefully, no extreme measures—I know because I overheard them talking with Dr. Seiler—but nothing is written in the chart. Dr. Anderson looked at the chart, and there is nothing: no silver sticker in the shape of a bullet, no initials for 'do not resuscitate.' Nothing was said to us. I wish I had let her go."

"Pauline, you did the right thing."

"Not right for her. For us. For Dr. Seiler and Dr. Anderson and for the hospital, but not for her. Aren't we here for the patient's good? Isn't that what we're *for*?"

"Not to make a decision like that."

"But the decision was made. I overheard it. It just wasn't written down."

"Then you can't be sure it was made. Listen, Pauline, do you know what I'm worried about? This will surprise you. I'm worried about Mrs. Culbertson being hand-bagged by someone who is not an R.N. Can you put an R.N. on her and send the L.P.N. back to the Shipley Wing?"

"That's Lonnie McDonough. She's the best we have, better than some R.N.'s. She's squeezing the handle of the bag, that's all. Mrs. Culbertson knows her—"

"I can't risk it, with this case."

"This case? Mrs. Culbertson is not a case. Don't you remember when you and I made a speech together for the fund drive at the Butterworth house by the ocean, and after the speech we had tea and the summer people talked to each other and Mrs. Culbertson sat next to me? She asked me why I became a nurse, and I told her my grandmother was a nurse and was so good to me I wanted to do whatever she had done. If she had been a streetwalker, I would have done the same thing. Mrs. Culbertson laughed at that and didn't even edge away. She said that when she was young, she went to Quebec to photograph the city buildings. The architecture of Quebec is special. Of course, I had never paid any attention to it. She told me that among her things she had a picture of my street—*my street!*—because she photographed a church there, and I said that must be my church. She would find the photograph and send it to me. And later she did, she *did*. I have it! Can you imagine? She didn't even edge away when she had a chance. I kept giving her a chance—"

"Pauline, do exactly what you are doing until you hear from Gerry."

* * *

Avis Markson stands in the long upper corridor, staring at the floor. Snow tracks have not discouraged her in the past— she has worked as housekeeper here for forty-four years—but this morning the tracks are grittier, the snow packed down harder into islands of immovable gray ice.

"Avis, I have a photograph."

She walks with me to my office, where Dr. Seiler is sitting in my chair. He doesn't move, and I ignore him. In the large brown envelope of photographs on my desk I find the one of Avis standing next to her cart laden with mops and pails. The floor beneath and behind her is a checkerboard of black and white tile, recently polished. It is a day after a snowstorm, and the afternoon sun, made brighter by the reflecting snow, shines through the glass doors at the far end of the hall and catches the brilliance of polish on the floor. The corridor stretches behind Avis and narrows to a gleaming point of light. In another fifteen minutes the hall will be tracked with the footprints of visitors. No matter, we have a photograph of the moment.

The phone rings. It is Dr. James saying that Dr. Hart, the anesthesiologist, has vanished.

"What do you mean *vanished*?"

"He is nowhere to be found."

"Where could he have gone?"

"Well, *I* don't know. You're the administrator of this so-called hospital, why don't you figure it out? You have no anesthesia backup and I have to cancel my case and I am plenty furious, let me tell you."

I should have made a point of talking more with Dr. Hart. He comes and goes without saying more than a subdued good morning and good-bye. His placid, wrinkled face holds no expression. He always arrives well in time for his first case, never late, moves carefully through each procedure, preparing his patients silently, watching and monitoring, writing his notes in the record in neat block letters—accurate, minimal, no more than is necessary. If only he would complain about something—his schedule, his fees, his contract—or behave like the others—barge into my office, pound on the desk and kick the walls, or shout through the telephone and send memos denouncing my complete lack of sensitivity to the needs of the medical staff—then I would feel comfortable with him, free to ask him questions. He and Dr. Wilmer are the only two anesthesiologists on staff. Dr. Wilmer left yesterday for a week's skiing. Can I get an anesthesiologist from a neighboring hospital? Not enough time. Change the medical staff bylaws to permit a nurse anesthetist? Over Dr. James's dead body. I call the operating room supervisor. Has someone checked his house? Yes. Who has cases booked today? Dr. James has already canceled his first two cases; Dr. Cartwright has a knee repair with the arthroscope at nine-thirty and a total hip replacement at noon; Dr. Johnson, a lens implant at ten in the small operating room; Dr. James again, a gallbladder for one-thirty. Four cases, down from six.

Dr. Seiler remains seated in my chair, expressionless.

"Well, you're beginning to dress better, I see. That brown velvet jacket, very nice. The board must have raised your salary."

"Art, how well do you know Dr. Hart?"

"So he's disappeared. Well, it fits."

"Why does it fit?"

"He keeps to himself, always has. The board brought him here twenty years ago, something about not being accredited by the Joint Commission if the anesthesiologist wasn't board-certified. I gave anesthesia then, no problems. But that wasn't good enough. Dr. Hart cut me out of a lot of business."

"Where is he likely to go?"

"Don't know anything about him."

"Who does?"

"Nobody."

"*Nobody?*"

Outside, the snow falls relentlessly, in larger and larger flakes.

"Father O'Malley."

I call Father O'Malley, and he says he will think and call me back. I ask him not to tell anyone about this. The word would spread through town—it takes less than an hour—that the hospital has no way of giving anesthesia and if you need surgery, you'd better get yourself over to Dover or Portland, even in snow, because this hospital can't keep its doctors in line. A story like that locks itself in. The rescue squads pick it up and take local patients to other hospitals. The story becomes fact in the minds of hundreds of people. To correct it takes months, years.

I call the police to report Dr. Hart's disappearance. I call Dr. Wilmer's ski resort to leave a message. I call the surgeons who have cases booked. It is an understatement to say that surgeons do not like the unexpected. I call the administrators of the nearest hospitals to tell them our situation and ask to speak to their anesthesiologists. Hospital administrators think in the possessive singular. My shop, my docs, my board. My anesthesiologists.

"Bill, listen, we can't find Dr. Hart, something may have happened to him, and my other anesthesiologist is away until Thursday. Would your doctors help us out? . . . Yes, I imagine you do have a full schedule. . . . Oh, yes, I know, but your Dr. Bell likes to come over here. He thinks small hospitals are fun—a zoo, he calls this one. . . . That's true, you could have a major emergency. . . . You don't mind if I call him, do you? . . . Okay, thanks. Bill, listen, what we all need is an anesthesia group to cover the whole region. Can we talk about it? . . . Okay, Bill, sometime. . . ."

If my shop loses patients, Bill's shop gains.

Bill and I meet often as members of a consortium of rural hospitals determined to cooperate—on group purchasing of supplies, laundry, perhaps an elevator repair contract—while remaining, of course, independent. If hospitals divided services among themselves ("you take obstetrics, we'll do orthopedic surgery"), they could reduce the cost to the public. But they would run smack into antitrust laws against restraint of trade. On medical matters, competition is strong.

On the other hand, if Maine should relax its antitrust legislation for hospitals, the Portland hospitals could get together and form a system. Would they draw us in or bury us?

I call Dr. Bell and leave a message.

Art Seiler gets up to leave. "Well, have fun," he says. He has in his hand a photograph of himself.

"Leave the picture, Art. It's going in the annual report."

"Just this one of me? Or all of the medical staff."

"All."

He pulls the photographs out of the envelope and spreads them on top of the desk. Twenty-three photographs of doctors. Large, eight by eleven, black and white.

"Looky here, our new cardiologist, Dr. Blankenship, why is he grinning? From a high-powered residency, too. What do you suppose he's doing *here*? Every time one of these turkeys comes begging through the door you smile and lay out the welcome mat and say, 'Why, yes, come in' "—his sugarcoated voice imitating mine—" 'we can certainly talk about staff privileges, and let me show you around our lovely town and invite you to my house and take you to dinner and introduce you to all the other doctors.' "

"We have an open staff."

"Well, it's time we close the gates. You're in over your head tampering with the pockets of physicians who were here holding up the walls of this hospital before you knew there was such a thing as a hospital administrator, which there wasn't back then, and we were better off."

"Decide what specialists we need. I have asked you for years to do that."

"We don't need any. Look here, Dr. Robert Fitzwater. What do we need with a gastroenterologist? You know what he's doing, of course you do, you're smart, you know everything, he and the cardiologist have multiple staff privileges, at Dover, at Biddeford, you name it. They see patients here on Wednesdays and lure them over to a bigger hospital, for convenience. Do you think they admit them here? Not on your life. Do you think they send a referred patient back to the family doctor? Hell, no, they don't. They're robbing you blind. And look at this, Dr. Grossmartin from Cleveland, a fancy-assed internist who specializes in rheumatology and 'likes the easygoing lifestyle of this charming town.' How is he going to make a living here? I have never seen a single case of rheumatoid arthritis."

"Never?"

"Never."

(Perhaps there haven't been any.)

"Maybe they will draw patients here from the county when

the word spreads." I wish I hadn't said that; it was a mistake. I gather up the photographs.

"Wait a minute. You're covering up Dr. Anderson. Now doesn't he look intelligent! He's taken thirty patients from me in one year. What am I supposed to do about that? You tell me."

"Take him in as a partner."

The phone rings. It is Dr. James. The fifteen-year-old with acute appendicitis needs surgery immediately.

"We have no anesthesia. Can we send her to Portland?"

Dr. James is patient. "Have you looked out the window? Nothing is moving."

I give the phone to Dr. Seiler. "Sounds like you have a decision to make."

Dr. James will do the case, with Dr. Seiler giving anesthesia. I say we can be sued up and down the pike if something goes wrong. He is halfway out the door, leaning back in.

"Not 'we,' *you*. This is an emergency. We, the medical staff, do the best we can with what *you* have provided." He looks almost pleased as he hurries off to the operating room.

I call Dr. Bell and leave a message giving him temporary privileges in anesthesia at this hospital beginning at 6:30 A.M. today; I make the same call to two anesthesiologists at two other hospitals; I dictate letters confirming my phone calls; I make written notes and place them in the file. In case something goes wrong. In case a suit is brought and it turns up in deposition that we were unable to meet the standard of medical care stated in our own bylaws that a board-certified anesthesiologist will provide anesthesia. We can blame his absence on the snow.

No sign of Eddie—it is 9:30 A.M. I call Nathan Barnstone, Eddie's uncle, manager of the shoe factory where Eddie works.

"No, haven't seen him. You say he's driving nurses in? Don't count on it. Oh, by the way, the big boss at headquarters wants me to renegotiate our managed care contract with you, says you no longer qualify as a preferred provider for our employees with the rates you charge, you and your doctors; we can do better with the group in Sanford. Unless you reduce your rates."

"Nathan, I can show you our costs—"

"Yeah, well, let me show you *my* costs, for health care benefits for employees. It's thirty percent. We have found a better deal."

"Wait. You could make a mistake going with the lowest bidder. You need to consider quality."

"If you had a measure for quality, then we would have something to compare. But you don't. None of you do, none of the hospitals in the state or anywhere else. We have to go by price. Our industry is up against foreign competition, shoes made in Korea, where labor is cheap. Do you know what Korean shoemakers work for? Ninety-five cents an hour. We can't compete with Far Eastern labor. Competition is killing us."

"Nathan, your employees *live* here. They've always come to this hospital, to these doctors. Have you asked *them*?"

"Yes, well, a letter is in the mail to you."

"Don't hang up. . . ."

The town dispatcher calls to say that all persons living on the coast are to be evacuated and sheltered in the high school gymnasium. The school will give them lunch. Can we provide dinner? Approximately ninety-four people. Yes. I call the kitchen.

"Annie, can you feed an extra ninety-four people tonight? Simple food, whatever you have."

"Feed the whole blooming town?"

"Mix things together, stretch what you have. You do it all the time."

"Like with twelve loaves and twelve fishes?"

"Something like that."

Three patients who were to be discharged this morning remain in the hospital without transportation. Carrie Williams is one. Carrie stands by the outside door in her coat and hat, holding a small suitcase. Bev Tracey holds her arm.

"Carrie, please do not try to walk home. It is not good weather."

Carrie starts out the door, Bev holding on to one arm and I the other. She shakes us off, saying we cannot legally detain her against her will. "Your house is too far," Bev says, "you could fall on the way, and no one would find you for hours. You could die in the snow by the side of the road!" Carrie walks out into the snow. Without coat or boots Bev walks behind her, trying to steer her back. Why does she want to leave? Have we been unkind, treated her badly? I follow.

"The collection," Carrie is saying. Her collection of china and glass at home, unguarded. She keeps on walking.

"Carrie, listen, my pitcher, we'll discuss a price."

Carrie stops. Bev gently turns her around to face the hospital. The three of us make our way slowly along the partially plowed driveway.

"Perhaps we can negotiate a deal."

"You liked the Lowestoft. Of course, it's priceless . . ." Carrie says as we push open the doors and enter the warm lobby.

Carrie has no money to pay for her heart medicine, which costs $67.90 for a week's supply. Unless she can sell her collection. But who will buy?

"Carrie, you are in for hard negotiations. Are you up to it?"

Pete is here. "We should postpone the noon meeting of the strategic planning committee and get through this day," Pete says. Snow is up to the top of the outside windowsills of my office and inching up the glass. Will it snow forever? Will we be cut off from light and air? Not a sign of Father O'Malley.

"Pete, we've postponed it twice this month because of one crisis or another. Today we will meet to discuss market share. From the latest figures we are losing the northwest and part of the northeast end of the county. We will not cancel this meeting."

"No one will be here."

"Then you and I will meet."

"Fine, let me show you the effect of the Maine Cost Review Board's cap on revenue . . ."

The revenue cap is based on an "average hospital." There is

no such thing. Every hospital in Maine is different from every
other. The state denies us our financial requirements.

". . . a four-hundred-thousand-dollar loss built into their
formula when applied to us. . . ."

At ten-thirty the state police found Dr. Hart by the side of
the Cage Road. He was sitting upright in the snow, wearing a
green and black plaid wool hat with all-around earmuffs, his
head resting against the slim trunk of a birch tree. The top of
his head was all the state trooper could see. The snow had
buried him above his eyes. The car lay upside down with its
four wheels still uncovered. The snow would have buried
them, too, in another hour.

"One-car accidents are usually suicide attempts," Jim Boze
says knowingly. He and Donny Whitworth got the ambulance
through and brought Dr. Hart to the operating room, where
Dr. James performed what amounted to, I learned later, open
heart surgery, a repair to the heart muscle. Dr. Seiler gave anesthesia. It was miraculous, the OR nurses told Gerry, who
told me—the ease with which Dr. James fixed the tear, well, it
was like standing next to Dr. De Bakey or someone who keeps
his hand in, she said, who like a natural hits a home run into
the lights and sends fireworks shooting through the sky, it was
that amazing.

"Close call. I'm sorry," Dr. Seiler says to me.

I lose control. "You're *sorry*? You ignored him for twenty
years because he took some income from you."

"What do you know? You weren't here."

"Cage talked to *you* when you came, told you all about the
flu epidemic. Talked to you even as you were stealing his patients. Couldn't you have done the same? He was lost. If we
can't be a place where even a doctor is kept from being lost,
then what can we be? I think we have blood on our hands."

"You are talking to *me* about this place? Are you committed here for life? Have you stood here for thirty years and
watched your practice erode and sift away from you and
watched others steal what was yours, piece by piece?"

"It's not *yours*, Art."

"Whose is it? Yours? A come-lately? You have no stake here, no history. You'll be gone in two years. Wanna bet?"

"Bet."

"Okay. Fifty bucks. Or better make it twenty-five. Your salary is probably a pittance, knowing these trustees. Jack Mathias told me you were the cheapest they could find."

Without missing a beat, I watch myself pick up the telephone, hear my own voice ask Dr. Bell to help us recruit an anesthesiologist.

Talk about *risk* when money is the only factor. . . .

Then I'm free to change my style, take risks, bet the shop.

Art Seiler is on his feet. "I am making rounds, walk with me."

We pass the nurse station, where Bev and Gerry are scheduling nurses for four hours' sleep and four hours' work starting with the three to eleven shift, until the snow stops. Still no sign of Eddie.

We stand at the door to room 11.

"Since your will is to know more . . ." Dr. Seiler mumbles in a voice so low I can barely hear him. He stands aside and lets me enter the room first. The lovely thin ghost face of Elizabeth Littlejohn lies on the white pillow. A man older than she sits in a chair by the bed.

"Get out!" Seiler shouts at the man. The man does not move. Dr. Seiler takes Elizabeth's wrist in his hand. "No food binges this time. Is this the porn king himself or just a flunky?" The man still does not move. "This pretty girl, this one here, drives her younger brothers and sisters over to Portland to a film studio—right, Elizabeth?—where they all pose for the cameras, don't they? Eh? Pretty good money in it for you, isn't that right? With all that money you don't have to live in your mother's dirt-floor shack with the kids crawling all over. You can rent a room from your grandfather, a whole room to yourself. I suppose this guy moved in with you. Is that why your grandfather threw you out?"

Elizabeth stares at Dr. Seiler with wide brown eyes, expressionless.

Dr. Seiler turns to me. "Will your famous chronic illness clinic solve Elizabeth's problems?" I say the clinic would include counseling. Dr. Seiler bursts out laughing and goes into one of his brief tap dance routines.

"Elizabeth," he says. "Ask this man to leave."

Elizabeth says nothing.

"Ask him to leave before I call the police."

Elizabeth turns her head to Dr. Seiler.

"It's snowing," she says.

The man gets up and walks out of the room. I watch him go down the corridor and out the door into the blinding snow.

Dr. Seiler pulls a chair up to Elizabeth's bed. All business now.

"I have requested a court order preventing you from visiting your brothers and sisters for one year. The Portland police are investigating the photographic studio and will want to talk to you. Your grandfather wants nothing to do with this, so we will keep you here until the whole thing is over. As a condition of your remaining here you will be required to see a counselor daily. Do you have any questions?"

Elizabeth shakes her head.

"Let us go on," Dr. Seiler says to me.

He leads the way down the corridor to room 7 and goes straight to the bed by the window where Ronald Flynn, a man in his sixties, with long gray-black hair and a week's stubble of beard, lies on top of the bed, still in his clothes, one leg exposed to the knee. A piece of shinbone rises from the leg into the air, protruding through the skin about three inches.

"Hello, Ronald, how is your leg?" Dr. Seiler slaps Ronald on the shoulder. "Ronald is a Christian Scientist. He doesn't want anything to do with conventional medicine, won't allow us to set his fracture properly, won't let the orthopedic doctor near him. Ronald, we could help that leg a lot if you would let us—"

Ronald shakes his head.

"Last night Ronald sprinkled Ajax cleaning powder all over his leg, to clean it, didn't you, Ronald?"

Ronald nods.

"Sure hope it doesn't get infected," Seiler says. "Infection wouldn't do that leg any good. Ronald won't take any medications, except morphine. He likes morphine a lot. Don't you, Ronald?"

Ronald nods again.

"Shouldn't we transfer him to a Christian Science sanatorium?"

"Ah. Indeed. I spent three hours on the phone last night calling to get him into one, but there is a problem. The problem is that Ronald is not a true member of the Church of Christ's Scientists, not a *card-carrying member,* you understand, so none of them will take him."

"So he stays with us."

"Bravo! Bravo! Hear it for the lady! She is catching on! Yes, indeed, she is!" Dr. Seiler shouts down the corridor. The nurses at the other end take no notice.

We go to room 6, a private room overlooking the river. A young man, about thirty, blond, with sunken cheeks and dark brown eyes staring out of some almost buried place, turns his head and reaches for a cigarette among the debris on his bedside table.

"Yeah, Doc?" Dr. Seiler lights a match for him. "I'm allowed to smoke because I'm dying," the man says to me. I shake his hand.

"My name is Kevin Hospice Littlejohn," he says, and beats on the bed with his empty hand, crinkles his eyes, and opens his mouth to laugh, but no sound comes, only a harsh breath, then swallowed air and a gasp from deep in his throat. He closes his mouth and smiles at me, watching to see if I get the joke, then looks at the white-haired lady sitting in the chair next to his bed. "I got hospice ladies round the clock. See, isn't she sweet? She listens to anything I tell her, and she tells me stuff when she feels like talking, and nobody pays her either. Says she's a volunteer. There's a bunch of them who sit here, like a watch, you know? the Black Watch, ha-ha. I forget your name, doll. What was it? Amanda Culbertson Greene? Yeah, how about that? Like having your own grandmothers. Yeah, Doc?"

"Yeah. How is the pain, Kevin?"

"Not bad. Listen, when I don't have no pain, does that mean I'm already dead and can't feel nothing?"

"No, it means the medicine I give you is working. You are by no means dead."

"Good, because Amanda here and I got something going. She's telling me a story that makes me wanna laugh, and I got to hear the end of it. She works for this hospice, see, not even paid, and they had a meeting last Friday, and half the group walked out of the room in the middle of the meeting and slammed the door. Amanda was one of them who walked out."

Amanda glances at me with a sheepish smile. Kevin throws his head back against the bed wallboard hangings of tubes and canisters and lets out a joyous roar—"Ahhhh-yaa"—and beats his hand on the bed. "*A work stoppage!*" he shouts, and then falls into a fit of gagging and coughing that lasts several minutes during which Dr. Seiler holds on to his shoulders and leans him over the basin while he spits blood.

"It was actually a protest," Amanda says in a subdued and serious tone, "against the direction in which our president is taking the hospice organization. She fails to understand the nature and spirit of hospice. It could be the end."

Dr. Seiler empties the basin in the sink and rinses it. Kevin lowers himself slowly into his pillows as if retreating into a secret world of his own.

"The end of what?" Dr. Seiler asks.

"You see, a group of us who know the town started a hospice, as a way of helping people who are . . . who need someone at a difficult time, and now this new faction says it should change to more than a group of volunteers. It should hire nurses and a social worker and become a business certified for Medicare payment."

"Oh, my." Art Seiler breathes a long sigh.

Kevin leans toward Amanda. "So what did you do after you slammed the door?"

"We tried to hear through the door, but Josie said there is a hole in the ceiling of the meeting room. Everybody knows about it. If you can get into the storage closet on the floor above, on some pretext, you can kneel down on the floor, turn yourself sideways, and stretch your ear to a certain opening in the corner from which you can hear most everything being said in the meeting room and can see, too, if you put your eye to it."

Kevin stares at Amanda. "You spied on the opposition?"

Amanda looks down. "Yes."

"Did you hear what they said?"

"Yes, one woman made a motion to ask us to come back, but no one seconded. Another woman said it was high time to lose the old guard. Hospice would draw in new members and proceed with a plan for the future. A younger person, who shall be nameless, described the mistakes our volunteers have made and would have talked on except that she looked up and saw me through the ceiling hole and gave a loud shriek, which broke up the meeting."

"She saw you? You were *caught*?" Kevin closes his eyes. "This could be the end after all."

Art Seiler stands near the door. "Are you coming?" he says to me.

"Wait," I say.

Kevin sits up, reaches for another cigarette. "Then what?"

"Well, I hurried home to think. In my embarrassment it was hard to think clearly. Eavesdropping is a serious infringement on the bounds of propriety, but in a desperate situation all tactics are legitimate. I called the members of our faction, and we agreed to meet then and there, to plan our next move. Within the half hour we gathered for lunch at the Stage Neck Inn. Eight of us were enough to form a separate hospice in the original spirit of service that brought us together in the first place, before the intrusion. We would begin again."

"Oh, fight, *fight*!" says Kevin.

Dr. Seiler is impatient. He breaks into a fox-trot and pulls Amanda to her feet. " 'Every day is ladies' day with me,' " he sings as he dances Amanda around and around.

"And with me," says Kevin. Amanda smiles and dances lightly. Kevin stubs out his cigarette and beats time with both arms on the bed.

In room 8 we visit Mary Gilford, who works at the Laundromat behind Rick's. Dr. James operated on Mary yesterday to repair a ruptured abdominal aortic aneurysm.

"Art, why wasn't this case transferred to Portland?"

"Should have been. James said he could handle it."

"*He* can handle it. We can't."

"She should be in intensive care. No room. Should I make a scene about it? I should. What good would it do? Six patients on this floor should be in intensive care. Pretty soon the whole hospital will be one big ICU. Put *that* in your strategic plan."

I know Mary's chances of recovery are not good after that kind of surgery.

A large young woman in thin pink trousers and a black leather jacket lies curled on the bed in a fetal position, resting on top of Mary's feet so that Mary, when she wakes, will feel a heavy weight on her feet as well as her abdomen. Bev Tracey joins us.

"She is Sally Gilford, Mary's daughter."

"Sally, come and sit in the chair," Dr. Seiler says. Sally sits up and hits him in the stomach with two hard fists. I hold one of her arms, and she twists it loose, grabs my hair, and pulls my head down hard against the bed rail, lies on the bed, shrieking that we are butchers and murderers, kicking Dr. Seiler and Bev with her feet weighted with snow boots, wrenching and struggling and screaming, finally on the floor, where Dr. Seiler holds her in a grip on both upper arms and I hold her legs. Bev grabs a pillow and puts it on the floor, and Seiler eases Sally down while Bev moves the pillow under her head. Dr. James comes in and steps easily over Sally to check on her mother. After a few minutes Sally sits up. We take her to the treatment room, where she slumps in the only chair and Dr. Seiler perches on the examining table. He says he will talk with her and I should wait for him in the intensive care unit.

In the unit Mrs. Culbertson's son Skip is with Pauline.

"Why did the nurses have to pound on her? Why couldn't they leave her alone? Who *are* these people? What is the matter with them?"

We wait for Dr. Seiler. When he comes, he walks past Skip to see Mrs. Culbertson, still on hand-bagged ventilation, Lonnie keeping an even stroke. He puts his fingers on her wrist, listens to her chest.

"You can stop now, Lonnie," he says.

"Didn't you tell them not to jump all over her like a pack of dogs? Didn't they *know*?"

"Know what, Skip?"

"Know enough to leave her alone, to let her go. It's what she wanted. . . . Yesterday I said that's what we wanted. Didn't you hear me?"

"You weren't sure. There was a doubt. You didn't know what you wanted. And your mother could not say what *she* wanted. She had a chance, you know; she could have recovered."

"Don't these nurses have any judgment?"

Pauline leaves the group.

"Did they hurt her?" Skip asks Dr. Seiler.

What can he say to this? *Of course they hurt her.*

Art Seiler takes a minute before he answers.

"When you were a kid, you liked those rocks at the far end of the beach. I used to see you from my boat. One time your mother brought you to my office bleeding with scrapes and cuts from climbing on the rocks. You had found a secret cave, and in it you felt like a pirate king who had discovered buried treasure. You said that, remember? Then you wanted to get out of the cave. While you were crawling through the narrow opening, a rock fell on you, bruised your neck, and cut the skin. Then you jammed for a minute in the opening before you saw you could get out by pressing your arms hard against the rocks. You pressed and it hurt, but you knew you were just about out onto the sand and were going to be okay. None of the bruises and scrapes bothered you much because you were out."

"You remember that?" Skip asks.

"Sure. I remember a lot."

Coleman lies at the apex of the half-circle wall in the intensive care unit. He has suffered a massive coronary. His arms are strapped to flat wooden splints wrapped with white gauze from wrist to elbow to keep the lines steady. There are lines everywhere: a line from a hanging IV bottle on his left dripping dopamine into his left arm; a needle installed in the top of his nose with a tube stretching back to the wall behind him; a line from below the sheet connected to an intra-aortic balloon pump inserted in the aorta which deflates and inflates at the appropriate times to increase or decrease the volume of blood in the heart; a line from his chest to an EKG machine. Even if he wants to, he cannot shift or turn himself without crossing wires. At least when he opens his eyes, he will see the river through the window.

"Coleman, don't answer, but if you could try to recover, I would be grateful because I am stuck."

Pauline asks me not to stay long.

I stand in stiff vigil staring at the green-line rhythm of Coleman's heart on the black screen, not frozen in panic but not able to move either. Am I surprised by illness? No. Am I useful? A wave of nausea comes over me. An unnecessary, undecorative, vestigial appendage, in the words of Art Seiler. Too old to go to medical school. Could I be a nurse? If I were a nurse, I would know whether the IABP apparatus had been set properly to regulate the blood flow to Coleman's heart; I would know what the green lines mean and could understand the mysterious peaks and valleys of electrical messages on the monitor, could make him comfortable, or at least try, could interpret the writing in the chart, know what drugs he is given, watch for error. If I were a nurse, Dr. Seiler would tell me in straight language what is going on with Coleman, speaking, if not with respect, at least without sarcasm, because my knowing what is going on would be of value to the outcome. And I would know whether or not Art Seiler intends to call a consult.

I look around the half room—at the beige-pink floor and walls, a restful color; at the black Formica "column," latest and most modern, standing from floor to ceiling free of the walls to hold on four sides its oxygen outlets and suction pumps and all the mechanical appurtenances of modern medicine, standing like a monument to itself, needing only (to be complete) a carved inscription of the name of each patient who has been wired to it; a visitor chair (only one because visitors are allowed in one at a time and asked not to linger) of maple frame with a rose tweed-upholstered seat and back, from the cheaper line of hospital furniture. We could save money on these chairs, said Jack Mathias, because a visitor to the intensive care unit is apt in his grief and fear to be tentative, to sit down very slowly, remain still, and not stay long, thus sparing the furniture excessive wear and tear. Jack has saving ways.

When Coleman opens his eyes, he will look toward the window, but he will not see the river, he will see only snow falling, so his eyes will turn back into the room. A pastel by John Shipley hangs on the wall opposite Coleman's bed: a picture of a long, dry road leading to an adobe house, in New Mexico, perhaps, or Arizona. The picture is soft, without contrast, a hint of sun but no heat. The road does not draw you along. The house does not invite you in. A person looking at the picture is left lying where he is. When Coleman wakes up, he will look at this picture. I take it down and put it where no one will trip over it. From the hall I borrow a print of Rembrandt Peale's "Rubens Peale with a Geranium" and hang it in place of the other painting. In this picture the artist's brother sits next to the first geranium seen in America. His hand holds the clay flowerpot, and his fingers touch the earth inside it.

Coleman is my friend; he is one of *ours*. Everything must be done for him. He must have the best. The very best.

He is awake now.

"One whole side of your market area is fish," he says.

"Fish. Yes. Are you hungry, Coleman?"

"No. The other side, farmers. If they want to do it all themselves, let them."

Coleman closes his eyes. I will do anything, go to any lengths, spare nothing to get the best treatment for him, the best in the nation, in the world, even. Pauline asks me to move out of the way.

Art Seiler walks by the room. I follow him down the hall.

"Art, where is the new cardiologist?"

"Where is he? How should I know? Do I know where people are every minute?"

"Is he available for consults?"

"Might be."

"Art, listen, you are a superb doctor, there is nobody better, you are my own doctor, but don't you think a consult with Dr. Blankenship on Coleman . . . It's complicated, isn't it? What I mean is, you have known Coleman for thirty-five years, his medical history, everything about him, how he responds to treatment, what his strengths are, so using that extraordinary knowledge together with a specialist who knows all the latest drugs and balloons, you would have the perfect medical team, Art, you see, you and the cardiologist, you have what he doesn't have, a thorough knowledge of the patient, and he has the latest technology, you can blend the two together, *this is what we are for,* Art, something unique because we are small, something only we can do because we know each other so well, put all the advantages of your relationship with the patient together with the latest medical know-how. Talk about quality! Your practice will be a model. I can see now the arrival here of groups of distinguished physicians and scholars of the type who advise government on health care policy, coming here to discuss your approach and examine your records for the outcomes, asking your advice and inviting you to speak to groups around the country."

Art Seiler says nothing. I have intruded into medicine. Unforgivable, even in April.

"See what you have here, Art, an advantage! You have time to exchange information. Extraordinary, this combination of a general practitioner, a specialist, and time. Rarely occurs in a medical center. I don't mean that no one talks to anyone in a medical center; that's not it at all. But the pace is more hurried. There is so much to find out about all those strangers. Coleman is not a stranger. You start the race from halfway around the track. What a leg forward! That is what years of office visits and friendship do for you. And consider the trust Coleman has in you. See it from his point of view, a man fallen among medical people who guard their knowledge carefully by making it mysterious to an outsider. I mean, if he is a pilot shot down in the Burma jungle who finds himself flat on a stretcher of knots and ropes carried by Burmese tribesmen, with you, their chief, leading the way, feeding him and treating his wounds, does he turn his head to ask for a map? Does he, at some crossing of jungle paths, ease over onto his shoulder and say, 'Wait! Look here, this path to the left is the one; there are no roots across it, and the light is brighter. Shouldn't we go that way?' You and your tribesmen would laugh at him without breaking a single stride in your progress along the path to the right. Does he protest? No. He doesn't know where he is. If he asks where he is, he receives an answer from you in a language he does not understand. So he doesn't ask. He lies back and watches the leaves above his head while his wounded body is carried stretched out and weightless through the complicated twisted jungle day after day. He marvels at the speed of his travel. Carrying such a burden of trust, Art—you must know how completely he trusts you—don't you have a responsibility to use the resources at hand? ... Use what we have, Jack Mathias tells me every day like a broken record. We have a cardiologist; why not use him? Too many specialists have spread to the hinterlands to make a living, but we can benefit. Use him like an unexpected gift, here by an act of grace, if you can bring yourself to look at it that way."

Dr. Seiler says nothing, nor does he look at me. Nothing to do now but stumble forward.

"Selectively add his information to yours. It's the perfect synergy. If I had a say in what we do as a nation, I would replace the large hospitals with two or three smaller ones just for this purpose, to blend information about people in neighborhoods and the way they live their lives. It would cost too much, of course. It costs too much to take care of our own."

Art Seiler walks to Coleman's bed. He writes in the medical chart. Silence. Coleman's eyes are on Art Seiler. It is time for me to leave.

A man waits in my office. Suit and tie.

"How did you get through the *snow*?"

"I always get through."

Hal Erk, "detail man" (a salesman with knowledge of pharmaceuticals) for a large drug manufacturer, sits in the chair that gives him the best straight view of the mailboxes in the hall where the doctors pick up mail and messages many times a day. A drug detail man's sales efforts are directed to doctors, who prescribe drugs.

"Listen, Erk, we have a patient who has no money, only a house and some china, who has to pay sixty-seven dollars and ninety cents for seven pills every week. What do you have to say about that?"

"I say it's a problem. We have problems, too. Like we spend billions on research—"

"—and development, spare me that one, Erk, and spare me the one about the future of medicine being a tiny pill lost in the palm of my hand. *Your firm makes a gross profit over the diseased bodies of my neighbors.*"

On my desk is a letter from a Boston law firm whose title carries across the top of its letterhead six fine WASP names thinly engraved in black and separated by commas except for the last two names, between which there is a delicate ampersand, followed by a dense list of partners and would-be partners covering two full columns on the top half of the page. The letter states that our hospital is named in a suit filed by Todhunter Ingersoll Brown III, who has suffered great pain and hardship because of our alleged negligence in treating him for a thorn from a rosebush lodged in his foot eight months ago, that Mr. Brown presented himself to our emergency room in the belief that the hospital would render proper treatment, that after treatment a piece of the thorn remained lodged in his foot, causing infection and requiring further surgery in Boston, which has incapacitated Mr. Brown, causing him personal and economic hardship.

Dr. James opens the office door. "I need to talk to you for a minute," he says. In an instant I know what is coming. "I will be leaving next month, for an appointment in general and vascular surgery at Memorial in Houston."

Without him . . .

"It doesn't work here for me, you know. There is no one on my level. The intellectual stimulation . . . well, it just isn't here. I think you understand."

I do, I do.

"Dr. James, listen, what do you need? Can we recruit a partner for you, someone on your level? You must know a brilliant surgeon who is ready for a quiet life by the sea? What equipment would you like? The laser, we'll buy it; we'll have a special fund drive just for your list, postpone all other capital items. What else do you need? Be patient with us; we can get things. Did you know that magnetic resonance imaging is available now in a mobile system, the whole thing bouncing and rattling along the road from Bangor in a big trailer truck—"

"Thanks, but no. Everything takes too long here. You see, in Texas I will have equipment at my fingertips. And more than that, I will have an appointment at the Veterans Administration Hospital also, and that means a research lab. The VA hospitals were generously overbuilt with government funds; they have extra space. And it means something else. I know you will understand this. The other day I saw a patient in my office. I have successfully operated on him twice, but there is an underlying condition, something I am not sure about that I want to follow, for my own knowledge, but the laboratory test is expensive. His insurance will not pay, and the patient cannot afford it. In the VA system I can order the test, and the system will pay without question, as long as I say the test is necessary. And it *is* necessary, for my own knowledge. Not that the man's treatment will change or that it will make any difference to his well-being. I simply want to know."

If I could drink enough coffee, I could stay up all night and write a grant application for a research project for Dr. James. Persuade Skip Culbertson to chair a special fund drive.

If I could . . .

"Without you we will be a second-rate hospital."

"No, you won't. Something will come to you."

As Dr. James leaves, Robert Butterworth III of the summer colony comes in. He spent the weekend here. Too much snow to drive back to Providence.

"Thought I'd let you know that some of us with cottages here are thinking of selling. It's getting congested in the summer with all the tourists. A large group of us knows about a quiet town, unspoiled—on the skids actually, prime property for sale at bottom price—where we can sort of have the place to ourselves in the summer. . . ."

"Where?"

"Down on the north shore of Massachusetts."

"Look, Mr. Butterworth, take a minute and consider. The working poor of this town have known you a long time. Remember how they have cleaned your cottages, served your cocktail parties, sold you lobster and corn, boarded your dogs, repaired your flagpoles, watered your geraniums? They know you well from the long years of remembering your grandfathers and grandmothers, great-aunts and uncles. Familiarity is a good thing; it eschews contempt. Not so much the money earned as the length of time passed that makes the difference. You might not find this elsewhere. Take time, consider. . . ."

What would keep the summer colony here? A better hospital, better equipped? The newest technology?

The lights go out. I count slowly to seven. Seven seconds, the length of time it should take for the emergency generator to turn on. . . . five, six, seven, eight. A dim half-light comes on in the hall. Out on the patient floor every third ceiling light is on. We are on emergency power.

"John Ferry, you are an extraordinary man."

He looks me straight in the eye. He has tested and polished his emergency generator daily for as long as he or anyone can remember, for one moment. Now.

"*I divorce you, I divorce you, I divorce you!*" Eddie Barnstone shouts at Bev in the corridor, stomping his boots and shaking snow all over. It is 2:00 P.M. He has brought in three nurses. Jeanie Seeger asks if she will be paid for the six hours she spent riding around in Eddie's Jeep while he lost his way in the snow over and over. I say yes, of course.

"Thank you, Eddie. Can you cook?"

Eddie stares at me.

"We need you in the kitchen."

Usually in the early afternoon I close the office doors and sleep for a few minutes with my head on the desk. Today I sleep for fifteen minutes—longer than usual, but I am dreaming and do not want to wake up. In my dream I am standing near the rocks on the far end of a small beach. It is summer. Under my feet is a square of sand fenced on all four sides without a gate. The sun is warm on my face. In the water there is a rowboat in which a woman sits quietly. The boat is drifting. The woman does not row; she is still, allowing the boat to drift wherever the current takes it. On the beach, standing together in a tight cluster, are Dr. Cage, Jack Mathias, Tony, John Shipley, Bev, Dr. James, Dr. Anderson, Charlene, Gerry, Dr. Talley, Art Seiler, Dr. Hart. Others. They are all there. They wave and call to the woman drifting in the rowboat. Coleman is in the boat—no, he is on the beach with the others. I am making a rope for them to throw to the woman, braiding it out of strips of green surgical linen and scraps of white three-by-five cards which I find on the ground, hurrying to put it together, but I cannot do it fast enough because my fingers are all thumbs. I know that if I do not work fast, the boat and the woman in it and all the people on the shore will disappear. Dr. Seiler and Jack Mathias call to me to hurry. Pete is picking up linen strips and counting as he hands them to me over the fence. We work fast but not fast enough, and the rope I am making unravels itself at one end as I braid the other. The tide is coming in. After a while I put my head down on the sand and fall asleep.

"The power is off in the high school. We are bringing all evacuees to the hospital." The voice of the town dispatcher comes over the telephone.

Donny Whitworth drives the ambulance from the high school to the hospital, carrying people evacuated from houses along the coast. He pulls up at the door, a Jeep and a pickup behind him. Through the heavy snowflakes, still coming down, I can see John Simpson, who is blind, and his ninety-two-year-old mother, coming through the door. Behind them are Harriet Blythe and her two sisters, climbing out of the pickup without hesitating, each as agile as the next, all three of them looking like Humpty-Dumpty dolls in barrel coats crowned with scarves and mufflers and decked in snowflakes, leaving only their eyes and noses exposed to the weather.

Art Seiler stands at the door, welcoming the evacuees as if greeting guests at a reception. Here are John and Eleanor Winslow and their four children and Eleanor's mother, Ruth Demar. Ruth stretches out two arms to Dr. Seiler.

"Oh, my dear doctor, you are wonderful to do this for us!"

Art Seiler straightens his tie and smooths the sleeves of his jacket. Coming in are Dan Appel, local contractor, and his two teenage boys, followed by Lindsay and Jean Webber and their six adopted children, all Vietnamese, and Lindsay's father and aunt, and behind them Gertrude McKinnon and her two boarders, one on each arm, very thin and fragile ladies of ninety or so, walking slowly, each step a careful undertaking, blocking the door. Behind them, jumping with impatience, Donny Whitworth's three young daughters and their mother, Sara. Dr. Seiler directs them to the cafeteria in the finest cruise director style, the best I have ever heard. "A lot of my paying patients are here," he says to me, with the look of a boy reeling in a splendid catch.

For dinner we have what the patients are having: canned cling peaches and red Jell-O and a soup Annie made with a delicious flavor of bay leaves. In it are many varieties of meat and vegetables. With the soup we eat salt-free crackers, which we unwrap from cellophane, two to a package. There is enough for everyone. Eddie Barnstone has made us a tuna delight out of macaroni and canned tuna topped with bright orange cheddar cheese melted and browned under the broiler.

Flora Littlejohn brings Gerry to the table where I sit, and we talk about Dr. Hart's recovery ("Out for three months"; "Rotate the OR nurses through his home care? No way"). Surrounded by a host of neighbors, we talk in low tones, unheard in the general noise of the cafeteria, about the suit against the hospital on behalf of Mr. Brown, who had a rose thorn in his foot ("Ask Charlene to talk to *no one* until our lawyer meets with her"), about Dr. James's departure, the death of Mrs. Culbertson, how to keep cans of Ajax away from Ronald, how to keep an eye on Carrie so she won't walk home, how to get through the night and then tomorrow with an exhausted staff. Eddie Barnstone sits on the floor in the corner, weeping quietly. Bev sits next to him and strokes his hair. John Ferry and his crew unfold cots, move tables and chairs to the other end of the cafeteria. In a minute we will have to move. Father O'Malley joins us. The telephone lines are dead, he says; we are cut off. Outside, beyond the cafeteria window, the snow continues to fall. It will cover us. We can shout and no one will hear. Buried and forgotten. I look for Hobart and his plow, but it is nowhere in sight.

TEN

The morning after the big snow, Fred Ames plows the driveway. The sky is hazy with the possibility of sun. Mountains of snow line the driveway and fill half the parking lot.

I am talking on the phone with Carolyn Roberts, president of Copley Hospital Systems in Morrisville, Vermont. She is a rural hospital expert with a national reputation. She will influence health policy.

"Community service is everything. The entrepreneurs in the hospital field are having trouble. People are the key. Match the hospital to the community . . ."

I have seen Copley Hospital—modest buildings on a large tract of land in a year-round community of small farms and businesses, more poor than rich. From the hospital a long driveway winds through a field to a frame building, a row of town houses designed to look like one large New England house. The field extends beyond the houses and is bordered by woods. Behind the woods are the Green Mountains. It is low-income housing for the elderly, separate units with a common room and a porch.

". . . with basic services. Decide what distance, time, and access to basic services should be; answer that; then develop the system that assures them."

"What about quality?"

"Quality measures are in their infancy, but innovative work is going on throughout the country. The Health Care Financing Administration's scorecard for hospitals has been nothing more than a list of hospital inpatient Medicare deaths compared with predicted deaths, based on *probability* according to diagnosis and condition. The more patients we send home or to nursing homes to die, the better it looks on the HCFA mortality list. But now we have to get at the real information on quality."

"What is the 'real' information?"

"Compliance with accepted clinical standards and patient satisfaction."

I am thinking of Miss Janssen. "One of our patients refused surgery and pain medication and died in the hospital, of lung cancer. An individual case. . . . By our quality assurance standards it was a preventable death."

At Copley a passageway leads from the main hospital to a large building for rehabilitation therapy. Most of the inside is one large room, a gymnasium. There is a sunlit square of space where an injured person can learn to walk again between parallel bars and up and down mock stairs, an alcove with a whirlpool bath, other alcoves for speech and hearing therapy, a section for learning (again) to use industrial equipment and ordinary kitchen devices—simple things like a faucet, a can opener made for one-hand operation, forceps, hand brushes, an oven temperature dial.

Copley is on the frontier. Basic service is fantastically innovative.

I talk to Paul Bengtson, chief executive officer of Northeastern Vermont Regional Hospital, in St. Johnsbury. He manages the hospital by contract. A firm specializing in central management of freestanding community hospitals, free of the local past, advises him.

Paul says: "With support of a full service contract, a manager can have more credibility when trying something new or when making a controversial recommendation."

Credibility. Yes. But cost is a factor. The hospital pays a fee for a management contract.

"The fee focuses the board's attention on performance," Paul says. "You balance the pros and cons of a contract. To the community it can mean admitting a need for help. Or it can mean a desire to do things better, depending on one's point of view. And when I need an outside resource, there is no confusion about where to find it."

No confusion . . .

The management firm gives Paul the necessary detachment to do the job. He is not overly distracted by contract issues. Instead, like any effective chief executive, he makes himself a valuable, useful member of the community.

I talk to Jud Knox, administrator of Camden Hospital, a small hospital competitively overshadowed by Penobscot Bay Medical Center down the road.

"Jud, are we all targets for closing?"

"No, not targets. Government policy does not say to close any size or type of hospital, just to shrink the system. The hospital system is fat. Reduce it, shrink it any way possible, let it fall out, let the chips fall where they may. That's what competition is for."

Jud is leaving Camden to become chief executive officer at another small, robust hospital on the Maine coast.

"What will be your strategy for survival?" I ask him.

"Look, if we think only about survival, we will fail. But if we try to be the best, we will survive. We have to advance but not by increments. Slow step-by-step building of programs won't save us. It will have to be a big move, a risky one, something really off the wall."

"What kind of move?"

"A new way of thinking. Right now we think in terms of our own convenience. Why is a waiting room called a *waiting* room? Because it is convenient to us to make the patient wait. Why do we plant ourselves indoors and *wait* for the patient to come to us? Instead a nurse goes into a home to preadmit a patient to the hospital. What patient wants to sit in a hospital lobby? A nurse visits an expectant mother before she delivers, then follows her home with the baby. Another nurse visits at other times, for routine care of well children. The motivation—

the incentive, if you like—is to keep people well. And our struggle, in the new order of things, will be to preserve relationships: doctor to patient, nurse to patient, hospital to community."

"Staff nurses leave the floors and fan out all over town?"

"When beds are empty, we send nurses home without pay. Makes them nervous. Wouldn't you be? Instead send them out where they are needed. I am talking about thinking. . . ."

Dear Gerry,

Your profession is ahead of its time. Long into the future, beyond feminism, nursing is the model for the new technological society. The more information you have, the more compassionate you become. What other profession can say that?

But building your future around the example of medicine could lead to danger. You could become an angry shadow. Specializing in one or another narrow field—do you think this is the road to status and professional autonomy? Why? Just because day after day you pick up the pieces dropped by physicians; because they are the hospital's customers (an unfortunate piece of jargon) who admit patients, or not, as they choose, to whom we cater right and left: We build their office buildings, buy their equipment, draw them in, in, in, to forge a common purpose? You could call it bribery. Some call it an exchange relationship of mutual benefit. (You will have noticed that in return physicians often hedge their own survival by setting up clinical labs and imaging centers in their offices, undercutting the hospital. Then the hospital retaliates by expanding ambulatory care, something physicians have taken for granted as their office territory. And so the war continues. It wastes precious energy and escalates the rising cost of medical care.)

Your own newly acquired visibility calls for a new strategy. The serious shortage of nurses has put you out in front, on everyone's mind. You had to disappear to be noticed.

Only the nursing profession knows how to be both specialized and broadly informed at the same time. A unique quality. It will make the difference in the chaos that is coming.

Only the nursing profession makes a specialty of drawing other professions together on behalf of a patient. Your talent for connection—in a disparate, fractured, conflicting multi-agency contrived-turf battleground health care system—is what makes American health care function as well as it does. Here we will change our definition of "status." It will have more to do with association, less with autonomy.

If a cardiac nurse worked in obstetrics, an operating room nurse in the slow time creep of the long-term care unit, an emergency room nurse in home care, the reduction effect on the budget would be monumental. But beyond that, usefulness expands geometrically by the kinds of information nurses can gather. I happen to have in my desk some three-by-five cards on which to begin a study (small, at first) of cause and effect. Yours is the only profession that does not discourage easily when health promotion fails and "prevention" programs appear to make no difference. Time and again I have watched you pick up the pieces and renew your own enthusiasm. Your staff is a research center waiting to happen because you follow your patients and link one piece of information with another, to see the end result of your work. You could dig in, draw closer; you are the friend physicians cannot be because of the weight they carry. You could fan out all over town. All it would mean is a mixed-up staffing schedule and fewer nurse committee meetings. Consider starting with the Littlejohn family. Then when the computer is up and ready for your data, you will publish your findings.

Your affinity—no, more than that, your *talent* for information is going to take care of us during the coming revolution in health care, which promises to be stormy. If it succeeds, your informed compassion will be the reason.

I need your ideas. They do not have to be new. There have been several good ones around on the fringe of health care for many years, and where are we if not on the fringe?

And something else. I am thinking about the internal organization of hospitals: self-perpetuating board, separate medical staff, high and dry management. For years I believed it to be the wrong mix. But it is what we have. To throw it out would waste almost a century of utility! Instead we will add a fourth group, consisting of nurses who will bring information from our neighbors. Then we will *have* something and can get started. The inevitable chaos does not worry me because you will be here keeping order, as you always have.

Please form a task force (I suggest Bev Tracey to lead) to decide what distance, time, and access to basic services should be, then develop the transportation system (mix together combinations of paid and volunteer drivers) that assures them.

Would you arrange a time on my calendar to discuss these matters?

In the living room of the Shipley Wing the light is good, and I can see the yellow tablet on which I am writing notes for a strategic plan. Carrie Williams is nearby. Her wheelchair is placed so that the late April sun shines on her lap, on the crocheted wool afghan of dazzling colors—deep sea blue and black, flamingo pink, tangerine, lemon, neon green, robin's egg blue. On a long table in front of her are stacks of cups and saucers, flowered and gold-bordered dinner plates, crystal, silver, American pewter. Everything on the table is for sale. Carrie has sold her house and car. When her collection is sold and all the money spent down, she will apply for Medicaid.

Mr. and Mrs. Butterworth look carefully at several sets of bone china.

"They're worth a fortune; she doesn't even know it," Mr. Butterworth says. "We've got the bargain of a lifetime."

Note: In an environment where greed nourishes itself at the public trough on behalf of its own ...

Tim Bailey stands for a moment in the doorway of the room staring at Carrie, then disappears.

... where in the shadows of a rich and powerful and immoral nation thirty-seven million people are without health insurance ...

"Tim used to sleep in my barn," Carrie says.

Art Seiler looks at everything on the table and writes a big check. He tells Carrie to pick out what his wife will like.

. . . and in a place where strengths and weaknesses—size, location, memory, a charitable base, usefulness, lifestyle, loyalty—are the same; where a weakness turns into a strength with a change in point of view (size, for instance, prohibits economies of scale but allows vigilance and attention) . . .

Dr. Wing, the new chief of surgery, talks with Carrie about the Lowestoft china, then decides on an American pewter bowl.

. . . some constraints are recognized: government programs fall short, private life alone does not sustain, communities must intervene. . . .

Jack Mathias stands in the doorway, staring at the room as if lost. Then he walks over to me.

"Selling china?"

"Jack, listen, you think this is off the wall, but you haven't seen anything yet."

(Manage *as if* backed by a contract.)

"Are we in some difficulty?" Jack asks.

"More than difficulty. This may be the end. No doubt we brought it on ourselves, in stubborn isolation, but I think we have been abandoned."

"By the enemy?"

"You disregard government, but government has no interest in *us* either. Health care is political, and if politics is the trading of property, what do we have to trade? Oh, now and then a congressional committee shows interest, in election years, and articles appear in the newspaper, and we are a big story for a few weeks, but it doesn't last. We have been abandoned, and when that happens in war—and this is war—when a company in combat finds itself lost, the officer gives the order to live off the land. 'Off the land' means use what we have, dig and fish for the rest, and I honestly believe that you, Jack, more than anyone else will find this congenial."

Considering the necessity of community intervention, a strategy is proposed: to adopt some features of a consumer cooperative, choosing directors by open democratic election—one citizen, one vote . . .

"Most elements of survival, Jack, like food, water, electricity, telephones, fire insurance, have gone to cooperatives at one time or another. To preserve access to basic necessities. Members join for their mutual benefit, giving the organization a staunch quality which makes up for your having to share control with your neighbors, whom I know you think of as your own."

"Too many people . . . you'll get into a fight."

"A New England fight. A return to democracy. Tony will join us; he knows about last-ditch efforts. You, Jack, will want to call on everyone in town with means above everyday poverty. John Shipley will watch from his window for the arrival of the summer people. Then your son, Phil, the marketing consultant, and Skip's nephew, Steve, the financial analyst, and Coleman's great-nephew, the strategic planner, all of the new innovative generation, can (that is, if elected by the membership) put their minds to the principles of mutual benefit. And as treasurer you will have to attend all meetings to fight every point. The meetings may stretch out . . . long afternoons, rich argument, a lot of interest. I hope you can sacrifice the time."

. . . *dues from the membership to help rebuild a charitable base, no patronage refunds.*

Dr. Anderson buys a fine cut glass vase.

Therefore, its being unlikely for members, who hire physicians and think of them as their own, to bring suit . . .

"Then with a strong base our local plan will nest congenially into the HMOs and regional cooperatives, networks, alliances, and systems of the enlightened state of Maine. They will seek us out."

. . . *and anticipating a new health care system achieved through a stunning symbol of the art of political compromise, we intervene, resisting discouragement in disease prevention and past failure of health promotion* . . .

Gerry and Bev buy a variety of cups and saucers in different patterns.

. . . *to configure the hospital for treatment of short-term illness, chronic and long-term care; to establish incentives and standards for community health; to include emergency care, family practice, surgery unrelated to volume, by competent*

*physicians seeking a lifestyle, by specialists selected accord-
ing to need based on open-system feedback on cause and effect, cost and quality; achieving—by public, community, and
private means—not exactly a profit but a contribution to the
future.*

John Shipley asks Carrie to accept a painting, one of his
own, of a boat shipwrecked in a storm at sea, as fair trade for
a set of plates. She tells John to hang the painting on the last
bit of wall space in the Shipley Wing. Then she asks John Ferry
to repair a cracked saucer. Tommy Littlejohn picks up a delicate teacup with the hook and clasp that takes the place of his
hand. He holds the cup high in the air, for a long minute, it
seems. No one speaks. He puts it down carefully. Tommy's
fiancée, Cassandra, buys a blue vase.

"What quality!" Skip Culbertson says out loud, addressing
the room.

Coleman walks in from the hall, pushing an IV pole on
easy-rolling steel casters. He makes a handsome offer for a
dozen bowls with a blue and gold band around the edge. I buy
my pitcher.

"Coleman, how long do you think it will take us to develop
and implement a strategic plan?"

"Decades."

"But we don't have decades!"

"No. On the other hand . . ."

Dear Tony,

The game is on!

A second chance.

On your way home from Florida would you put your
mind to the matter of reinventing the hospital? The old in-
tractable institution will give way to one where new ideas
are manageable.

We will carve out a local design—health care is still a local matter—then set it up, measure its usefulness, move it
out for display, and publish our findings.

What small hospitals can contribute to the national debate is this: Because they have no margin for error, they
know themselves well, stay close to home, remember the

best and worst of their past, weigh what they can and cannot do, and pay attention. There is a lot to be said for them.

This is an opportunity, Tony, for quality.

It could turn out to be the catbird seat.

No doubt you have already drawn circles around it.

Looking forward to your return.

Rex McCullough flies around the racetrack corridor of the Shipley Wing in his sleek world-class sports wheelchair, past his slower-moving elderly neighbors, then streaks with perfect timing through the doors of the living room. He wears sunglasses and a silk scarf. One fast roll of the wheels, and he is across the room and parked in his spot between the two bookcases.

"Where did he come from? How long will he stay?"

"He has spina bifida, unusual in a thirty-five-year-old. A feisty, energetic man, always arguing."

"He causes havoc, wheeling too fast, crashing into people in the corridor."

Sara Woodson of the Women's Auxiliary hurries in and shuffles among sheet music near the piano. She adjusts the bench and sits down, flexing her fingers in preparation. The room is almost full now with patients and nurse's aides and volunteers. Two Auxiliary ladies in pink smocks—newcomers from away, I do not recognize them—sit together at the desk in the corner.

Father O'Malley makes Carrie an offer for a tall Dresden coffeepot. Carrie does not look up. She looks straight into the sun-brilliant colors of the blanket on her lap, moving only to put her thumb through one of the holes in the crocheted pattern. Not a hole, exactly; more like a carefully designed space between one complicated knot after another.

"You'll have to do better than that," she says.

As the singing begins, Father O'Malley writes on a piece of paper, adding figures, taking his time, each time subtracting and refiguring. Carrie shakes her head and hands back the paper. Their voices rise and fall; they gesture, glare, turn their

backs. Father O'Malley walks out of the room. When he returns, they will begin again.

"Carrie, you drive a hard bargain."

"Are we stuck here for this songfest?"

"Yes."

Astute, compassionate, and written with tremendous subtlety, Susan Garrett's portrait of a small hospital in Maine offers compelling insight into just how inseparable human interest is from the politics of health care. In the tradition of such masters as Annie Dillard and John McPhee, Garrett uses careful and graceful personal descriptions to shed light on major issues.

This hospital is a place where doctors, nurses, and staff know every patient's name, stay overtime to help when a neighbor is admitted, and pitch in during blizzards. They struggle with rising costs, expensive high-tech medicine, Medicare regulations, and other contemporary health-care challenges that threaten to close it down. As Susan Garrett looks at a year in the life of this community hospital and tells its true story, she fills it with history, sharp observations, amusing anecdotes, daily drama, and glimpses into the private lives of medical personnel, trustees, staff, and patients. And her fascinating, wise narrative becomes a microcosm of what's gone wrong, what's stayed right, and what's truly needed in today's medicine.

Susan Garrett worked as the administrator of this hospital, located in three red-brick buildings on a hill near the rocky Maine seacoast; her life became inextricably entangled in its daily battles between quality health care and cost. She tells us about: searching for beds for the uninsured and homeless...Dr. James, the hospital's star surgeon and main money-maker, who threatened to leave if the hospital refused his demands for ever more expensive equipment...Carrie, the proud Yankee spinster, who must sell her heirlooms to pay for outrageously costly heart medicine...a summer of chaos in the emergency room...keeping the peace

MACBETT

OTHER WORKS BY EUGÈNE IONESCO
PUBLISHED BY GROVE PRESS

The Colonel's Photograph and Other Stories

Exit the King

Four Plays (The Bald Soprano; The Lesson; The Chairs; Jack, or the Submission)

Fragments of a Journal

Hunger and Thirst and Other Plays (The Picture; Anger; Salutations)

The Killer and Other Plays (Improvisation, or The Shepherd's Chameleon; Maid to Marry)

Notes and Counternotes: Writings on the Theater

Present Past, Past Present: A Personal Memoir

Rhinoceros and Other Plays (The Leader; The Future Is in Eggs)

A Stroll in the Air and Frenzy for Two or More

Three Plays (Amédée; The New Tenant; Victims of Duty)

MACBETT

A PLAY BY
EUGÈNE IONESCO

Translated from the French
by Charles Marowitz

GROVE PRESS, INC.
NEW YORK

PERFORMANCE NOTICE

Macbett was first performed on January 27, 1972 at the Théâtre de la Rive Gauche in Paris.

The English language premiere was performed by the Yale Repertory Theatre in New Haven, Connecticut on March 16, 1973. It was directed by William Peters, John McAndrew and Alvin Epstein; music composed by Gregory Sandow; sound by Carol M. Waaser; scenery design by Enno Poersch; lighting design by Ian Rodney Calderon; costume design by Maura Beth Smolover; and with the following cast:

MACBETT	Alvin Epstein
DUNCAN	Eugene Troobnick
LADY DUNCAN	
LADY MACBETT	Carmen de Lavallade
FIRST WITCH	
SECOND WITCH	
LADY IN WAITING	Deborah Mayo
MAID	Amandina Lihamba
GLAMISS	John McAndrew
CANDOR	William Peters
BANCO	
MONK	Stephen Joyce
MACOL	
BISHOP	Michael Gross

PERFORMANCE NOTICE

SOLDIERS, GENERALS,
BUTTERFLY HUNTER,
GUESTS, CROWD,
LEMONADE SELLER,
ETC.

} Josepha G. Grifasi
Michael Gross
Amandina Lihamba
John McCaffrey
Paul Schierhorn
Michael Quigley

MACBETT

A field.

GLAMISS *and* CANDOR. GLAMISS *enters from left as* CANDOR *enters from right.*

They come on without acknowledging each other and stand center stage, facing the audience.

Pause.

GLAMISS (*turning toward* CANDOR) Good morning, Baron Candor.

CANDOR (*turning toward* GLAMISS) Good morning, Baron Glamiss.

GLAMISS Listen, Candor.

CANDOR Listen, Glamiss.

GLAMISS This can't go on.

CANDOR This can't go on.

GLAMISS *and* CANDOR *are angry. Their anger and derision become more and more emphatic. One can hardly make out what they're saying. The text serves only as a basis for their mounting anger.*

3

GLAMISS (*derisively*)   Our sovereign . . .

CANDOR (*ditto*)   Duncan. The beloved Archduke Duncan.

GLAMISS   Yes, beloved. Well beloved.

CANDOR   Too well beloved.

GLAMISS   Down with Duncan.

CANDOR   Down with Duncan.

GLAMISS   He hunts on my land.

CANDOR   For the benefit of the State.

GLAMISS   So he says . . .

CANDOR   He *is* the State.

GLAMISS   I give him ten thousand chickens a year and their eggs.

CANDOR   So do I.

GLAMISS   It may be all right for others . . .

CANDOR   But not for me!

GLAMISS   Me neither.

CANDOR   If they're prepared to take it, that's their business . . .

GLAMISS   He's drafting my men into his army.

CANDOR   The National army.

GLAMISS   Sucking me dry.

CANDOR   Sucking us dry.

GLAMISS   Taking my men. My army. Turning my own men against me.

CANDOR   And me.

GLAMISS   Never seen anything like it.

CANDOR   My ancestors would turn over in their grave . . .

GLAMISS   So would mine!

CANDOR   And there's all his cronies and parasites.

GLAMISS   Who fat themselves on the sweat of our brow.

CANDOR The fat of our chickens.

GLAMISS Of our sheep.

CANDOR Of our pigs.

GLAMISS Swine.

CANDOR Of our bread.

GLAMISS Ten thousand chickens, ten thousand horses, ten thousand recruits. What does he do with them? He can't eat them all. The rest just goes bad.

CANDOR And a thousand young girls.

GLAMISS We know what he does with them.

CANDOR Why should we owe him? It's he who owes us.

GLAMISS More than he can pay.

CANDOR Not to mention the rest.

GLAMISS Down with Duncan.

CANDOR Down with Duncan.

GLAMISS He's no better than we are.

CANDOR Worse, if anything.

GLAMISS Much worse.

CANDOR Much much worse.

GLAMISS Just thinking about it makes my blood boil.

CANDOR It really gets me worked up.

GLAMISS My honor.

CANDOR My glory.

GLAMISS Our ancestral rights.

CANDOR My property.

GLAMISS My land.

CANDOR Our right to happiness.

GLAMISS He doesn't give two hoots.

CANDOR He doesn't give one!

GLAMISS We're not nobodies.

CANDOR Far from it.

GLAMISS We stand for something.

CANDOR   We're not just "things."

GLAMISS   We're nobody's fool—least of all Duncan's. Ha, beloved sovereign!

CANDOR   He won't lead me up the garden path or sell me down the river.

GLAMISS   Sell me up the river or lead me down the garden path.

CANDOR   Even in my dreams.

GLAMISS   Even in my dreams he haunts me like a living nightmare.

CANDOR   We must get rid of him.

GLAMISS   We must get rid of him—lock, stock, and barrel.

CANDOR   Lock, stock, and barrel.

GLAMISS   We want freedom.

CANDOR   The right to make more and more money. Self-rule!

GLAMISS   Liberty.

CANDOR   Running our own affairs!

GLAMISS   And his!

CANDOR   *And* his!

GLAMISS   We'll split it between us.

CANDOR   Half and half.

GLAMISS   Half and half.

CANDOR   He's a lousy administrator.

GLAMISS   He's unfair!

CANDOR   We'll establish justice.

GLAMISS   We'll reign in his stead.

CANDOR   We'll take his place.

CANDOR *and* GLAMISS *walk toward each other. They look stage right, where* BANCO *enters.*

CANDOR   Hail Banco, gallant general.

GLAMISS   Hail Banco, great captain.

BANCO   Hail Glamiss. Hail Candor.

GLAMISS (*aside to* CANDOR)   Not a word about you-know-what. He's loyal to Duncan.

CANDOR (*to* BANCO)   We were just going for a little stroll.

GLAMISS (*to* BANCO)   Very warm for this time of year.

CANDOR (*to* BANCO)   Would you like to sit down for a moment?

BANCO   No thanks. I'm taking my morning constitutional.

GLAMISS   Ah yes. Very good for your health.

CANDOR   We admire your courage, you know.

BANCO   I do my best for King and Country.

GLAMISS (*to* BANCO)   Quite right, too.

CANDOR   You're doing a grand job.

BANCO   Now gentlemen, if you'll excuse me. (*He goes out left.*)

CANDOR   Farewell, Banco.

GLAMISS   Farewell, Banco. (*To* CANDOR) We can't count on him.

CANDOR (*half drawing his sword*)   He's got his back turned. We could kill him now if you like. (*He tiptoes several paces toward* BANCO.)

GLAMISS   Not yet. The time isn't ripe. Our army is unprepared. We need more time. It will be soon enough.

CANDOR *sheathes his sword.* MACBETT *enters stage right.*

CANDOR (*to* GLAMISS)   Here's another of the Grand Duke's loyal subjects.

GLAMISS Hail Macbett.

CANDOR Hail Macbett, faithful and virtuous gentleman.

MACBETT Hail Baron Candor. Hail Baron Glamiss.

GLAMISS Hail Macbett, great general. (*Aside to* CAN-
DOR) He mustn't suspect anything. Act natural.

CANDOR Glamiss and I are great admirers of your
fidelity, your loyalty toward our beloved sovereign,
the Archduke Duncan.

MACBETT Why shouldn't I be faithful and loyal? After
all, I took the oath of allegiance.

GLAMISS No, that's not what we meant. On the contrary, you're quite right. Congratulations.

CANDOR His gratitude no doubt is very satisfying.

MACBETT (*with a broad smile*) The generosity of King
Duncan is legendary. He always has the good of the
people at heart.

GLAMISS (*winking at* CANDOR) Quite right, too.

CANDOR We're sure he does.

MACBETT Duncan is generosity incarnate. He gives
away all he possesses.

GLAMISS (*to* MACBETT) You must have done quite
well by him.

MACBETT He's also brave.

CANDOR Great exploits testify to his courage.

GLAMISS It's common knowledge.

MACBETT He's everything they say he is. Our sovereign is good, he's loyal, and his wife, our queen, the
Archduchess, is every bit as good as she is beautiful.
She is charitable. She helps the poor. She tends the
sick.

CANDOR How could we not admire such a man?—A
perfect man. A perfect ruler.

GLAMISS   How could we not be loyal in the face of such loyalty? How could we not be generous amidst such generosity?

MACBETT (*almost suiting the action to the word*)   I'd fight to the death against anyone who said the contrary.

CANDOR   We're convinced, absolutely convinced, that Duncan is the most virtuous ruler the world has ever known.

GLAMISS   He is virtue itself.

MACBETT   I do my best to follow his example. I try to be as courageous, virtuous, loyal, and good as he is.

GLAMISS   That's not easy.

CANDOR   Because he's a very good man indeed.

GLAMISS   And Lady Duncan is very beautiful.

MACBETT   I do my best to resemble him. Farewell, gentlemen. (*He goes off left.*)

GLAMISS   He almost convinced me, for a minute.

CANDOR   He's a believer. A . . . .

GLAMISS   He's incorruptible.

CANDOR   A dangerous character. He and Banco are the commanders-in-chief of the Archduke's army.

GLAMISS   You're not trying to back out, are you?

CANDOR   No—certainly not. I don't think so.

GLAMISS (*hand on his sword*)   Just don't try it, that's all.

CANDOR   No, I won't. I really won't. Yes, yes, of course you can count on me. Of course, of course! Of course!

GLAMISS   Right. Let's get a move on then—polish our weapons, gather our men, prepare our armies. We shall attack at dawn. Tomorrow evening Duncan will be beaten and we shall share the throne.

CANDOR   You do believe Duncan's a tyrant, don't you?

GLAMISS   A tyrant, a usurper, a despot, a dictator, a
miscreant, an ogre, an ass, a goose—and worse. The
proof is, he's in power. If I didn't believe it, why
should I want to depose him? My motives are thoroughly honorable.

CANDOR   I suppose you're right.

GLAMISS   Let's swear to trust each other completely.

CANDOR *and* GLAMISS *draw their swords and salute
each other.*

GLAMISS   I trust you and I swear on my sword to be
absolutely loyal.

CANDOR   I trust you and I swear on my sword to be
absolutely loyal.

They sheathe their swords and go out quickly,
GLAMISS *to the left,* CANDOR *to the right.*

*Pause. The stage is empty. Great play should be made
here with the lighting on the cyclorama and with sound
effects, which eventually becomes a sort of musique
concrète.*

*Shots are fired. Flashes. We should see the ripple of
gunfire. A conflagration in the sky on the backcloth.*

*Equally a very bright light could come from above
which would be reflected off the stage. Storm and lightning.*

*The sky clears. A beautiful red sky on the backcloth.
A tragic sky. At the same time as the horizon clears,
and turns red, the sounds of machine-gun fire become
more and more infrequent and fade into the distance.*

Shouts, death rattles, the groans of the wounded are heard—then more shots. A wounded man screams shrilly.

The clouds clear. A large deserted plain. The wounded man stops screaming. After two or three seconds' silence a woman's shrill scream is heard.

This should go on for a long time before the characters in the next scene appear. The lighting and the sound effects should have nothing naturalistic about them— especially toward the end. The contributions of the lighting designer and sound technicians are of crucial importance here.

Toward the end of the sound track, a SOLDIER *fences his way across the stage from left to right—flourishes, lunges, salutes, corps a corps, feints, direct attacks, all sorts of parries.* All this happens quickly.

The noises stop for a while before beginning again. Silence. The flourishes, etc., happen quickly. There should be nothing balletic about them.

A woman, disheveled and weeping, runs across the stage from left to right.

The LEMONADE SELLER *enters stage right.*

LEMONADE SELLER Lemonade. Cool and refreshing. Soldiers and civilians, buy my lovely lemonade. Roll up, roll up. Who wants to wet his whistle? There's a truce on. Better make the most of it. Lemonade, lemonade. Cure the wounded, lemonade to keep you from getting frightened. Lemonade for soldiers. One franc a bottle, four for three francs. It's also good for scratches, cuts, and bruises.

TWO SOLDIERS come on from left. One is carrying the other on his back.

LEMONADE SELLER (*to the* FIRST SOLDIER) Wounded?
SOLDIER No. Dead.
LEMONADE SELLER Sword?
SOLDIER No.
LEMONADE SELLER Bayonet?
SOLDIER No.
LEMONADE SELLER Pistol shot?
SOLDIER Heart attack.

The TWO SOLDIERS go out right.

LEMONADE SELLER Lemonade. Cool and refreshing. Lemonade, for soldiers. Good for the heart. Good for the shakes. The willies. The heebeejeebees.

ANOTHER SOLDIER enters right.

LEMONADE SELLER Refreshing drinks.
SECOND SOLDIER What are you selling?
LEMONADE SELLER Lemonade. It heals wounds.
SECOND SOLDIER I'm not wounded.
LEMONADE SELLER Keeps you from getting scared.
SECOND SOLDIER I'm never scared.
LEMONADE SELLER One franc a bottle. It's good for the heart as well.
SECOND SOLDIER (*tapping his breastplate*) I've got seven under here.
LEMONADE SELLER Good for scratches, too.

SECOND SOLDIER   Scratches? I've certainly got a few of those. We fought long and hard. With this. (*He shows his club.*) And this. (*He shows his sword.*) But especially with this. (*He shows his dagger.*) You shove it in his belly . . . in his guts. That's the part I like best. Look, there's still some blood on it. I use it to cut my bread and cheese with.

LEMONADE SELLER   I can see well enough from here.

SECOND SOLDIER   Scared, are you?

LEMONADE SELLER (*terrified*)   Lemonade, lemonade. Good for stiff necks, colds, gout, measles, smallpox.

SECOND SOLDIER   I killed as many of 'em as I could. Mashed 'em up something horrible. They yelled and the blood spurted. What a do! It ain't always as larky as that. Give me a drink.

LEMONADE SELLER   It's on the house, general.

SECOND SOLDIER   I'm not a general.

LEMONADE SELLER   Major.

SECOND SOLDIER   I'm not a major.

LEMONADE SELLER   You soon will be, though. (*Gives him a drink.*)

SECOND SOLDIER (*after several gulps*)   Revolting. Cat's piss. What a nerve. It's daylight robbery.

LEMONADE SELLER   You can have your money back.

SECOND SOLDIER   You're shaking. You're scared. It doesn't stop you getting the shakes, does it? (*He draws his dagger.*)

LEMONADE SELLER   Don't do that—please.

A bugle call.

SECOND SOLDIER (*sheathing his dagger and going off left*)   Lucky for you I haven't got time. But just you wait. I'll get to you again.

1 3

LEMONADE SELLER (*alone, trembling*) Whew, he really scared me. I hope the other side wins and cuts him up into little pieces—minced meat and mashed potatoes. Bastard. Swine. Shithead. (*Change.*) Lemonade, lemonade. Cool and refreshing. Three francs for four.

He goes out right slowly at first, then gradually getting quicker as the SOLDIER, *with his sword and dagger, re-appears stage left.*

> *The* SOLDIER *catches the* LEMONADE SELLER *just as he's going off into the wings. All we can see, in profile or from behind, is that the* SOLDIER *strikes the* LEMONADE SELLER, *and we hear him cry out. The* SOLDIER *disappears as well.*

> *The noise of shooting, screams, etc. begins again, but softer now, further away. The sky flares up again, etc.*

> MACBETT *enters upstage. He is exhausted. He sits down on a milestone. In his hand is a naked sword. He looks at it.*

MACBETT   The blade of my sword is all red with blood. I've killed dozens and dozens of them with my bare hands. Twelve dozen officers and men who never did me any harm. I've had hundreds and hundreds of others executed by firing squad. Thousands of others were roasted alive when I set fire to the forests where they'd run for safety. Tens of thousands of men, women, and children suffocated to death in cellars, buried under the rubble of their houses which I'd blown up. Hundreds of thousands were drowned in the Channel in desperate attempts to escape. Millions died of fear or committed suicide. Ten million others died of anger, apoplexy, or a broken heart. There's not enough ground to bury them all. The bloated bodies of the dead have sucked up all the water from the lakes in which they throw themselves. There's no more water. Not even enough vultures to do the job. There are still some survivors, can you imagine? They're still fighting. We must make an end of it. If you cut their heads off, the blood spurts from their throats in fountains. Gallons of blood. My soldiers drown in it. Battalions, brigades, divisions, army corps with their commanders, brigadiers first, then in descending order of rank, lieutenant-generals, major-generals and field marshals. The severed heads of our enemies spit in our face and mock us. Arms shorn from their trunks go on brandishing their swords and firing pistols. Amputated feet kick us up the backside. They were all traitors, of course. Enemies of the people—and of our beloved sovereign, the Archduke Duncan, whom God preserve. They wanted to overthrow him. With the help of foreign soldiers. I was right, I think. In the heat of battle, you often lay about you indiscriminately. I hope I didn't kill any of our friends by mistake. We were fighting shoulder to shoulder. I hope I didn't tread on their toes. Yes, we're in the right. I've come to rest awhile on this stone. I'm feeling a little queasy. I've left Banco in sole command of the army. I'll go and relieve him in a bit. It's strange— in spite of all this exertion, I haven't got much of an appetite. (*He pulls a large handkerchief out of his pocket and mops his brow and the rest of his face.*) I thrashed about a bit too hard. My wrist aches. Luckily it's nothing serious. It's been quite a pleasant day, really. Feeling quite bucked. (*He shouts to his orderly, stage right.*) Go and clean my sword in the river and bring me something to drink.

The ORDERLY *enters and goes out with the sword. He comes back immediately, without having completely left the stage.*

ORDERLY   One clean sword and a jug of wine.

MACBETT *takes the sword.*

MACBETT   Good as new.

He sheathes the sword and drinks from the jug of wine, while the ORDERLY *goes out left.*

No. No regrets. They were traitors after all. I obeyed my sovereign's orders. I did my duty. (*Putting the jug down.*) It's good, this wine. I'm quite rested now. Well, back to the grind. (*He looks upstage.*) Here's Banco. Hey. How's it going?

BANCO *or his* VOICE   They're just about retreating. Take over from me, will you? I'm going to take a bit of a breather. I'll join you in a bit.

MACBETT   We mustn't let Glamiss escape. I'll go and surround them. Quickly.

MACBETT *goes off upstage.* MACBETT *and* BANCO *resemble each other. Same costume, same beard.*

BANCO *enters right. He is exhausted. He sits down on a boundary stone. In his hand is a naked sword. He looks at it.*

BANCO The blade of my sword is all red with blood. I've killed dozens and dozens of them with my own hand. Twelve dozen officers and men who never did me any harm. I've had hundreds and hundreds of others executed by the firing squad. Thousands of others were roasted alive when I set fire to the forests where they'd run for safety. Tens of thousands of men, women and children suffocated to death in cellars, buried under the rubble of their houses which I'd blown up. Hundreds of thousands were drowned in the Channel in desperate attempts to escape. Millions died of fear or committed suicide. Ten million others died of anger, apoplexy or a broken heart. There's not enough ground to bury them all. The bloated bodies of the dead have sucked up all the water from the lakes in which they threw themselves. There's no more water. Not even enough vultures to do the job. There are still some survivors, can you imagine? They're still fighting. We must make an end of it. If you cut their heads off, the blood spurts from their throats in fountains. Gallons of blood. My soldiers drown in it. Battalions, brigades, divisions, army corps with their commanders, brigadiers first, then in descending order of rank, lieutenant-generals, major-generals and field marshals. The severed heads of our enemies spit in our face and mock us. Arms shorn from their trunks go on waving swords or firing pistols. Amputated feet kick us up the backside. They were traitors, of course. Enemies of the people—and of our beloved sovereign, the Archduke Duncan, whom God preserve. They wanted to overthrow him. With the help of foreign soldiers. I was right, I think. In the heat of battle, you often lay about you indiscriminately. I hope I didn't kill any of our friends by mistake. We were fighting shoulder to shoulder. I hope I didn't tread on their toes. Yes, we're in the right. I've come to rest awhile on this stone. I'm feeling a little queasy. I've left Macbett in sole command of the army. I'll go and relieve him in a bit. It's strange—in spite of all this exertion I haven't got much of an appetite. (*He pulls a large handkerchief out of his pocket and mops his brow and the rest of his face.*) I thrashed about a bit too hard. My wrist aches. Luckily it's nothing serious. It's been quite a pleasant day, really. Feeling quite bucked. (*He shouts to his orderly, stage right.*) Go and clean my sword in the river and bring me something to drink.

> *The* ORDERLY *enters and goes out with the sword. He comes back immediately, without having completely left the stage.*

ORDERLY   One clean sword and a jug of wine.

> BANCO *takes the sword.*

BANCO   Good as new.

> *He sheathes the sword and drinks from the jug of wine, while the* ORDERLY *goes out left.*

No. No regrets. They were traitors after all. I obeyed my sovereign's orders. I did my duty. (*Putting the jug down.*) It's good, this wine. I'm quite rested now. Well, back to the grind. (*He looks upstage.*) Here's Macbett. Hey. How's it going?

MACBETT *or his* VOICE They're just about retreating. Come and join me and we'll finish them off.

BANCO We mustn't let Glamiss escape. We'll surround them. I'll be right with you. (BANCO *goes out upstage.*)

The sounds of battle well up again. The conflagration in the sky is brighter now.

Pounding brutal music.

A woman crosses the stage from left to right. She is quite unconcerned and has a basket over her arm as if she were going shopping.

The sound dies away again until it is little more than a background murmur.

The stage is empty for a few moments, then ridiculously lavish fanfares drown out the noise of battle.

An OFFICER *in Duncan's army comes on quickly from the left and stops stage center. He is carrying a sort of armchair or portable throne.*

OFFICER Our lord, the Archduke Duncan and the Archduchess.

> LADY DUNCAN *and the* ARCHDUKE *come on left.* LADY DUNCAN *is in front of the* ARCHDUKE. *She is wearing a crown and a long green dress with a flower on it. She is the only character in the play who dresses with a certain flair.* DUNCAN *mounts the throne. The two others stand on either side of him.*

OFFICER   Come on, my lord. It's all right. The battle has moved on. We're out of range here. Not even a sniper about. Don't be afraid. There are even people strolling about.

DUNCAN   Has Candor been defeated. If so, have they executed him? Have they killed Glamiss as I ordered?

OFFICER   I hope so. You should have looked a bit more closely. The horizon is all red. It looks as if they're still at it, but a long way off now. We must wait till it's over. Be patient, my lord.

DUNCAN   What if Macbett and Banco have been routed?

LADY DUNCAN   You take the field yourself.

DUNCAN   If they've been beaten, where can I hide? The king of Malta is my enemy. So is the emperor of Cuba. *And* the prince of the Balearic Isles. And the kings of France and Ireland, and what's more, I've got lots of enemies at the English court. Where can I hide?

OFFICER   It's all right, my lord. You just leave it to Macbett and Banco. They're good generals—brave, energetic, skilled strategists. They've proved their worth time and again.

DUNCAN   I don't seem to have much choice. In any case I'm going to take one or two precautions. Saddle my best horse, the one who doesn't kick, and get my launch ready, the most stable vessel on the seven seas, the one with all the lifeboats. If only I could give orders to the moon—make it full, and order the stars to come out. For I really should travel by night. That's the safest thing. Safety first, I always say. I better bring a little money along, just in case. But where shall we go? Canada perhaps, or the United States.

OFFICER   Just wait a little while. Don't lose heart.

A WOUNDED SOLDIER *staggers on.*

DUNCAN   What's that drunk doing here?

OFFICER   He's not drunk. He's wounded.

DUNCAN   If you come from the battle, give me a report. Who's won?

SOLDIER   Does it matter?

OFFICER   Who's won? Was there a winner? You're in the presence of your king.

DUNCAN   I am your sovereign—the Archduke Duncan.

SOLDIER   Oh, I'm sorry, sir. I'm a bit wounded. I've been stabbed and shot. (*He staggers.*)

DUNCAN   It's no good pretending to faint. Answer me! Was it them or us?

SOLDIER   I'm not sure. It all got a bit too much for me. To tell you the truth, I left early. Before the end.

DUNCAN   You should have stayed.

OFFICER   Then he wouldn't be here to answer your questions.

DUNCAN   He left "before the end" as if it was a boring play.

SOLDIER   I fell down. Passed out. Came round again. Got up as best I could and, as best I could, dragged myself here.

DUNCAN (*to the* SOLDIER)   Are you sure you're one of ours?

SOLDIER   Who do you mean, "ours"?

OFFICER   The Archduke's and the Archduchess's, of course. They're standing right here in front of you.

SOLDIER   I didn't see you on the battlefield, my lord.

DUNCAN (*to the* SOLDIER)   What were your generals' names?

SOLDIER   I don't know. I was just coming out of the pub and a sergeant on horseback lassoed me. My mates were lucky. They got away. I tried to resist, but they hit me over the head, tied me up and carried me off. They gave me a sword. Oh, I seem to have dropped it somewhere. And a pistol. (*He puts the pistol to his head and pulls the trigger.*) Out of ammunition. Must have fired it all. There were a load of us out there on the field and they made us shout "Long live Glamiss and Candor."

DUNCAN   Traitor, you're one of our enemies.

OFFICER   I shouldn't cut his head off if I were you, my lord. Not if you want to hear the rest.

SOLDIER   And then they shot at us, and we shot at them.

DUNCAN   Who's "they"?

SOLDIER   And then they took us prisoner. And then they told me if you want to keep a head on your shoulders, you'd better join us. They told us to shout "Down with Candor, down with Glamiss." And then we shot at them and they shot at us. I was hit several times, wounded in the thigh, and then I guess I fell down. Then I woke up and the battle was still going on a long way away. There was nothing but heaps of dying men all around me. So, as I said I started walking; and my right leg is hurting, and my left leg is hurting, and I'm losing blood from the wound in my thigh. And then I got here . . . That's all I've got to say—except that I'm still bleeding. (*Gets up painfully. Totters.*)

DUNCAN   This idiot's made me none the wiser.

SOLDIER   That's all I've got to say. I don't know any more.

DUNCAN (*to* LADY DUNCAN)   He's a deserter.

LADY DUNCAN *draws her dagger. Her arm is poised to stab the* SOLDIER.

SOLDIER   Oh, don't bother yourself ma'am. (*He gestures off right.*) I'll just crawl over to that tree there and kick off. You can save yourself the trouble. (*He goes staggering off, left.*)

LADY DUNCAN   At least he's polite. Unusual for a soldier.

From the right, the noise of a body falling.

DUNCAN (*to the* OFFICER)   Stay here and defend me. I may need you. (*To* LADY DUNCAN) Quickly, take one of the horses, trot up to the front, then come back and tell me what's going on. Don't get too near though. I'll look through my telescope.

LADY DUNCAN *goes out right. While* DUNCAN *is looking through his telescope, we can see* LADY DUNCAN *upstage on her horse. Then* DUNCAN *folds up his telescope.*

Meanwhile, the OFFICER *has been standing with his sword drawn, looking menacingly in all directions.* DUNCAN *goes out right followed by the* OFFICER *carrying the armchair.*

Scene: near the battlefield.

Shouts of "Victory! Victory! Victory! . . ." coming from downstage left and right.

The word "victory" is repeated, modulated, orchestrated until the end of the following scene.

Sound of a horse galloping closer and closer is heard from the wings right. An ORDERLY *hurries on left.*

ORDERLY (*shading his eyes*) Is that a horse? I think it's coming nearer. Yes. It's coming toward us at full tilt.

BANCO (*comes on from left and shades his eyes*) I wonder what the rider wants, galloping so fast on that magnificent stallion. It must be a messenger.

ORDERLY It's not a man. It's a woman.

> *Sound of neighing. The hoof beats stop.* LADY DUNCAN *appears, a riding crop in her hand.*

BANCO It's her Highness, the Archduchess, the Archduchess. I humbly greet your highness. (*He bows, then kneels to kiss the Archduchess's hand.*) What is your Highness doing so near the battlefield? We're proud and happy that your Highness takes such an interest in our silly squabbles. As for our own life, we hold it at a pin's fee, but we are worried about your Highness's safety.

LADY DUNCAN Duncan has sent me for news. He wants to know what's going on and whether you've won the war.

BANCO I understand his impatience. We *have* won.

LADY DUNCAN Bully for you. Rise, my dear Macbett.

BANCO   I'm not Macbett. I'm Banco.

LADY DUNCAN   Excuse me. Rise, my dear Banco.

BANCO   Thank you, madam. (*To the* ORDERLY) What are you gaping at? Get the hell out of here, you stupid bastard.

ORDERLY   Yessir. (*He disappears.*)

BANCO   I apologize for that momentary indiscretion. Swearing like a trooper. Please forgive me, your Highness.

LADY DUNCAN   Of course I forgive you, Banco. It's to be expected in wartime. People are more high strung than in peacetime, obviously. The main thing is to win. If a few rude words are going to help the war effort, that's fine by me. Have you taken Baron Candor prisoner?

BANCO   Of course.

LADY DUNCAN   And Baron Glamiss?

MACBETT'S VOICE (*coming from the left*) Banco. Banco. Where are you? Who are you talking to?

BANCO   To her Highness, Lady Duncan, sent by the Archduke himself to gather information. Macbett will tell you about the fate of Glamiss.

MACBETT (*still offstage*)   I'll be right with you.

BANCO   I'll leave you to Macbett, madam. He'll tell you what's happening to our prisoners and give you a full account.

MACBETT'S VOICE (*quite near now*)   I'm coming.

BANCO   Excuse me, your Highness. I must go and feed my men. A good general is like a mother to his troops. (*He goes out left.*)

MACBETT'S VOICE (*nearer still*)   Coming. Coming.

MACBETT *enters left. He greets* LADY DUNCAN.

MACBETT   We have served our beloved sovereign well. Candor is in our hands. We've pursued Glamiss to a nearby mountain which you can see in the distance there. He's surrounded. We've got him trapped.

LADY DUNCAN   So you're General Macbett, are you?

MACBETT   At your command, your Highness.

LADY DUNCAN   I remember you looking different. You don't look very much like yourself.

MACBETT   My face looks different when I'm tired and I'm afraid I don't look very much like myself. People often take me for my twin brother. Or for Banco's twin brother.

LADY DUNCAN   You must get tired quite a lot.

MACBETT   War isn't a picnic. But one must learn to take the rough with the smooth. Let's say it's . . .

> LADY DUNCAN *puts her hand to* MACBETT *who kneels and kisses it, then gets up quickly.*

. . . an occupational hazard.

LADY DUNCAN   I'll go and tell the Archduke the good news.

BANCO'S VOICE (*in the wings*)   All clear.

> LADY DUNCAN *goes to the wings stage right and signals with her hand. She returns center stage. Fanfares are heard.*

MACBETT   His Highness the Archduke!

SOLDIER   His Highness the Archduke!

BANCO'S VOICE   The Archduke!

LADY DUNCAN   Here comes the Archduke!

BANCO'S HEAD (*appearing and disappearing*)   The Archduke!

SOLDIER   The Archduke!
MACBETT   The Archduke!
LADY DUNCAN   Here comes the Archduke!
BANCO'S VOICE   The Archduke!
SOLDIER   The Archduke!
MACBETT   The Archduke!
LADY DUNCAN   Here comes the Archduke!
BANCO'S HEAD   The Archduke!
SOLDIER   The Archduke!
MACBETT   The Archduke!
LADY DUNCAN   Here comes the Archduke!

> *Blazing fanfares. The sound of cheering.* DUNCAN *enters right. The fanfares stop.*

LADY DUNCAN   The battle is over.
MACBETT   Greetings, your Highness.
BANCO'S HEAD   Greetings, your Highness.
SOLDIER   Greetings, your Highness.
MACBETT   My humble greetings.
DUNCAN   Did we win?
MACBETT   The danger is over.
DUNCAN   Thank God. Has Candor been executed?
MACBETT   No, my good lord. But we've taken him prisoner.
DUNCAN   Why haven't you killed him? What are you waiting for?

MACBETT   Your orders, my good lord.
DUNCAN   You have them. Off with his head. Jump to it. What have you done with Glamiss? Have you torn him limb from limb?
MACBETT   No, my good lord. But he is surrounded.

Any moment now we'll take him prisoner. There's no cause for alarm, your Majesty.

DUNCAN   Well then, well done. I can't thank you enough.

The SOLDIERS *and the crowd shouting "Hurrah!" We don't see them—unless they're projected onto the back.*

MACBETT   We're proud and happy to have been of service, my good lord.

BANCO'S HEAD (*appearing and disappearing*) We were only doing our duty, my good lord.

More fanfares which get softer and softer until they become a background accompaniment to the scene.

DUNCAN   Thank you, my dear generals, and thank you, my gallant soldiers, who saved my country and my throne. Many of you laid down your lives in the struggle. Thank you all again, dead or alive, for having defended my throne . . . which, of course, is also yours. When you return home, whether it be to your humble villages, your lowly hearths, or your simple but glorious tombs, you will be an example to generations to come, now and in the future and, better still, in the past; they will keep your memory alive for hundreds and hundreds of years, in word and deed, voiceless perhaps but ever present, in fame or anonymity, in the face of an undying yet transient history. Your presence, for even though absent you

will be present to those who, whether they can see you or not, shall gaze lovingly at your photographs—your presence will serve as a pointer, tomorrow, and in the future, to all those who are tempted not to follow your example. As for the present, continue as you have done in the past, to earn your daily bread as gallantly as ever by the sweat of your brow, neath the sun's burning rays and under the watchful eye of your lords and masters who love you despite yourselves and whatever your shortcomings have a higher opinion of you than you might imagine. You may go.

Fanfares and hurrahs fainter now.

MACBETT   Bravo!
SOLDIER   Bravo!
DUNCAN   Nicely put, don't you think?
LADY DUNCAN   Bravo, Duncan! (*She applauds.*) That was a marvelous speech.

MACBETT *and the* SOLDIER *applaud.*

BANCO'S VOICE   Bravo!
DUNCAN   They deserved it. In future, my generals and my friends will all share in my glory. And my noble wife. (*He smiles at* LADY DUNCAN *and kisses her hand.*) You can all be proud of yourselves. And now, justice and retribution. Bring in Candor. Where's Banco?
MACBETT   He's with the prisoner.
DUNCAN   He will be the executioner.

MACBETT (*aside*)   That honor should have been mine.

DUNCAN   Let him approach with the traitor. Go and get him.

The SOLDIER *goes out left. At the same moment* CANDOR *and* BANCO *come on right. Banco's head is covered in a hood. He is wearing a red pullover and carrying an axe.* CANDOR *is handcuffed.*

DUNCAN (*to* CANDOR)   You're going to pay for your treachery.

CANDOR   And pay dearly. I have no illusions. If only I had won. The victor is always right. *Vae victis.* (*To* MACBETT) If you'd fought for me, I'd have rewarded you well. I'd have made you a duke. And you, Banco, I'd have made you a duke, too. You'd both have been loaded with honor and riches.

DUNCAN (*to* CANDOR)   Don't worry. Macbett will be Baron Candor. He'll inherit all your lands, and your wife and daughter, too, if he likes.

MACBETT (*to* DUNCAN)   I'm faithful to you, my lord. I'm faithfulness personified. I was born faithful to you, as a dog or horse is born faithful to its master.

DUNCAN (*to* BANCO)   Don't you worry, either. You've no need to be jealous. Once Glamiss is captured and beheaded, you will be Baron Glamiss and inherit all his property.

MACBETT (*to* DUNCAN)   Thank you, my lord.

BANCO (*to* DUNCAN)   Thank you, my lord.

MACBETT (*to* DUNCAN)   We would have been faithful.

BANCO (*to* DUNCAN)   We would have been faithful.

MACBETT   Even if you hadn't rewarded us.

BANCO   Even if you hadn't rewarded us.

MACBETT   Serving you is its own reward.

BANCO   Serving you is its own reward.

MACBETT   But as it is, your bounty well satisfies our natural greed.

BANCO   We thank you from the bottom of our heart.

MACBETT *and* BANCO (MACBETT *drawing his sword and* BANCO *brandishing his cleaver*)   . . . from the bottom of our heart. We'd go through Hell for you, your gracious Majesty.

A MAN *crosses the stage from left to right.*

MAN   Rags and bones! Rags and bones.

DUNCAN (*to* CANDOR)   You see how devoted *they* are?

MACBETT *and* BANCO   It's because you are a good king, generous and just.

MAN   Rags and bones! Rags and bones. (*He goes out left. The rag-and-bone* MAN *can be cut or kept in as the director wishes.*)

As he goes out, a SERVANT *comes in carrying armchairs for* DUNCAN, LADY DUNCAN *and the others.*

During the action which follows, he will bring a towel, a basin, and some soap, or perhaps just some eau de cologne for LADY DUNCAN, *who washes her hands—very emphatically, as if trying to get rid of a spot or stain. She should do this in a rather mechanical absent-minded way. Then the same* SERVANT *brings in a table and tea service and serves cups of tea to those present.*

The lights come up on a guillotine, and then gradually a whole forest of guillotines comes into view.

DUNCAN (*to* CANDOR) Have you anything to say? We're listening.

They all settle down to look and listen.

SERVANT (*to* LADY DUNCAN) Tea is served, madam.

CANDOR If I'd been stronger, I'd have been your anointed king. Defeated, I'm a traitor and a coward. If only I'd won. But History was against me. History is right, objectively speaking. I'm just a historical dead end. I hope at least that my fate will serve as an example to you all and to posterity. Throw in your lot with the stronger. But how do you know who the stronger is, before it comes to the crunch? The masses should keep out of it until the fighting is over and then throw in their lot with the winner. The logic of events is the only one that counts. Historical reason is the only reason. There are no transcendental values to set against it. I am guilty. But our rebellion was necessary, if only to prove that I'm a criminal. I shall die happy. My life is an empty husk. My body and those of my followers will fertilize the fields and push up wheat for future harvests. I'm a perfect example of what not to do.

DUNCAN (*quietly to* LADY DUNCAN) This is too long. Aren't you bored? I bet you're excited to see what happens next. No, no, we won't torture him. Just put him to death. Disappointed? I've got a surprise for you, dear. The entertainment will be more lavish than you thought. (*To everybody*) Justice demands that the soldiers of Candor's army be executed along with him. There aren't very many of them.

137,000—not too many, not too few. Let's get a move on. We want to be done by dawn.

Upstage a large red sun slowly sinks. DUNCAN *claps his hands.*

Go on. Off with his hea .
CANDOR   Long live the A: chduke!

BANCO *has already ar anged his head on the guillotine. To do so he has iad to get rid of his ax.*

One after another, CAI DOR's *soldiers pass in a continuous procession to the guillotine. (The same actors follow each othe around.)*

Another way to do it w ild be to have the scaffold and the guillotine appec as soon as DUNCAN *gives the order.* BANCO *pushe: the button and the heads fall.*

BANCO   Hurry, hurry, hurry, hurry!

After each "Hurry" the blade falls. The heads pile up in the basket.

DUNCAN (*to* MACBETT)   Have a seat next to my dear wife.

MACBETT *sits down beside* LADY DUNCAN. *They both need to be clearly visible so that the audience can see what's going on. For example,* LADY DUNCAN *and the others could be sitting with their backs to the guillotine but still appear to be watching the executions.* LADY DUNCAN *is counting heads.*

During the whole of this, the SERVANT *is serving tea to one or other of the characters, offering them buns and so on.*

MACBETT   I'm overwhelmed, madam, to be so close to you.

LADY DUNCAN (*still counting*)   Four, five, six, seven, seventeen, twenty-three, thirty-three, thirty-three— I think I missed one.

Without ever stopping counting, she starts nudging MACBETT *and playing footsy with him—at first discreetly, then more and more obviously until the whole thing becomes excessive and grossly indecent.*

MACBETT *edges away a little. At first he is rather embarrassed and confused. Then gradually, half-frightened, half-pleased, he gives in, eagerly acquiescing.*

DUNCAN (*to* MACBETT)   Now, back to business. I create you Baron Candor. Your comrade Banco will be Baron Glamiss when Glamiss has been executed in his turn.

LADY DUNCAN (*still fondling* MACBETT)   A hundred and sixteen, a hundred and eighteen, what a moving sight.

MACBETT   I'm very grateful to your Highness, my lord.

LADY DUNCAN Three hundred. I'm getting dizzy. Nine thousand three hundred.

DUNCAN (*to* MACBETT) Now listen carefully.

> MACBETT *disentangles himself a little from* LADY DUNCAN, *who continues to play with him, rubbing up against him and putting her hand on his knee.*

MACBETT I'm all ears, my lord.

DUNCAN I shall keep half of Candor's lands and half of Glamiss's too. They will be added to the crown estates.

LADY DUNCAN Twenty thousand.

BANCO (*still working the guillotine*) Thank you, your Highness.

DUNCAN (*to* MACBETT) There are some things you will have to do for me—both of you—in return. Certain duties, certain obligations, certain taxes to be paid.

> An OFFICER *runs onstage and stops center stage.*

OFFICER Glamiss has escaped!

DUNCAN I'll tell you the details later.

OFFICER My lord, Glamiss has escaped.

DUNCAN (*to the* OFFICER) What?

OFFICER Glamiss has escaped. Part of his forces rallied to him.

> BANCO *stops guillotining and comes downstage. The other characters jump up.*

BANCO How could he have escaped? He was surrounded. He was as good as taken. It's a conspiracy.

DUNCAN Damn!

LADY DUNCAN (*still pressing against* MACBETT) Damn!

MACBETT Damn!

DUNCAN (*to* BANCO) Whoever is responsible, you won't be Baron Glamiss nor get half his lands till you bring him before me bound hand and foot. (*Turning to the* OFFICER.) And you're going to have your head cut off for bringing us such disagreeable news.

OFFICER It's not my fault.

A SOLDIER *drags the* OFFICER *upstage to the guillotine. The* OFFICER *yells. They cut his head off.*

Music. DUNCAN *goes out.* LADY DUNCAN *plays footsy with* MACBETT *and rolls her eyes at him.*

DUNCAN *comes back on. The music stops.*

He addresses LADY DUNCAN *who is going out backward blowing kisses to* MACBETT.

DUNCAN Come along, madam. (*He drags her off by the scruff of the neck.*)

LADY DUNCAN I wanted to see what was going to happen next.

DUNCAN'S VOICE (*to* BANCO) Bring me Glamiss—by tomorrow.

Music.

BANCO (*going over to* MACBETT) We've got to start all over again. What a disaster.

MACBETT   What a disaster.
BANCO   What a disaster.
MACBETT   What a disaster.

Wind and storm.

The stage is dark. All we can see is Macbett's face—and the faces of the FIRST AND SECOND WITCHES *when they appear.*

Enter MACBETT *and* BANCO

MACBETT   What a storm, Banco. Terrifying. The trees look as if they're trying to pull themselves up by the roots. I just hope they don't topple onto our heads.
BANCO   It's ten miles to the nearest inn and we haven't got a horse.
MACBETT   We didn't realize how far we'd come.
BANCO   And now we're caught in the storm.
MACBETT   Still, we can't stand here all day discussing the weather.
BANCO   I'll go and stand by the road. Perhaps a cart will come along and give us a lift.
MACBETT   I'll wait for you here.

BANCO *goes out.*

FIRST WITCH   Hail Macbett, thane of Candor.
MACBETT   You frightened me. I didn't know there was anybody there. It's only an old woman. She looks like a witch to me. (*To the* WITCH) How did you know I'm thane of Candor? Has rumor added it's

murmur to the rustling of the forest? Are wind and storm echoing the news abroad?

SECOND WITCH (*to* MACBETT)   Hail Macbett, thane of Glamiss.

ʼ ᴀCBETT   Thane of Glamiss? But Glamiss lives. Besides, Duncan promised his title and his lands to Banco. (*He notices that it was the* SECOND WITCH *who spoke.*) Another one.

FIRST WITCH   Glamiss is dead. Drowned. The torrent swept him and his horse away.

MACBETT   Is this some kind of joke? I'll have your tongues cut out, you old hags.

FIRST WITCH   Duncan is very displeased with Banco for letting Glamiss escape.

MACBETT   How do you know?

SECOND WITCH   Duncan wants to take advantage of this. He is going to give you the title and keep the lands for himself.

MACBETT   Duncan is loyal. He keeps his promises.

FIRST WITCH   You will be Archduke and rule the country.

MACBETT   You're lying. I'm not ambitious. Or rather my only ambition is to serve my king.

FIRST WITCH   You will be king yourself. It is ordained. I can see the star on your forehead.

MACBETT   It's impossible. Duncan has a son, Macol, who's studying at Carthage. He is the natural and legitimate heir to the throne.

SECOND WITCH   There's another son who's just finishing a post-graduate degree in economics and navigation at Ragusa. He's called Donalbain.

MACBETT   Never heard of him.

FIRST WITCH (*to* MACBETT) You can forget about him. He won't interfere. (*To the* SECOND WITCH) It wasn't navigation. It was business studies—though obviously shipping was part of the course.

MACBETT Rubbish. Die. (*He waves his sword and strikes at the air. We hear the Witches' terrifying laughter.*) Hellish creatures.

They have disappeared.

Did I really see them and hear them? They've changed into the wind and storm. Disappeared into the roots of trees.

FIRST WITCH (*now a woman's melodious voice*) I'm not the wind. I'm not a dream, Macbett. I'll soon be back. Then you'll know my power and my charm.

MACBETT Jumping catfish! (*He takes three or four more swipes, then stops.*) I thought I recognized that voice. Who can it be? Voice, have you a body? Have you a face? Where are you?

FIRST WITCH (*melodiously*) Right beside you. Right beside you. And a long way off. Farewell, Macbett. Till we meet again.

MACBETT I'm shivering. It must be the cold. Or the rain. Or is it fear? Or horror? Or some mysterious longing that this voice arouses in me? Am I already under its spell? (*Change of tone.*) Filthy hags. (*Change of tone.*) Banco. Banco. Where can he have got to? Have you found a cart? Where are you? Banco. Banco. (*He goes out right.*)

Pause. The stage is empty. Noise of the storm.

FIRST WITCH (*to the* SECOND WITCH) Here comes
Banco.

SECOND WITCH When they're not together, they're
either following each other about or looking for each
other.

> The FIRST WITCH *hides stage right. The* SECOND
> WITCH *hides stage left.* BANCO *enters upstage.*

BANCO Macbett. Macbett. (*He makes a show of looking for* MACBETT.) Macbett, I've found the cart. (*To
himself*) I'm soaked to the skin. Luckily, it's slack-
ening off a bit.

> In the distance a voice calling "Banco."

I thought I heard him calling. He should have stayed
here. He must have got tired of waiting.

VOICE Banco! Banco!

BANCO Here I am. Where are you?

VOICE (*nearer now, coming from the right*) Banco!
Banco!

BANCO Coming. Where are you? (*He runs stage
right.*)

ANOTHER VOICE (*different, coming from the left*)
Banco!

BANCO Where are you?

FIRST WITCH'S VOICE Banco!

BANCO Is that Macbett?

SECOND WITCH'S VOICE Banco!

BANCO It doesn't sound like him.

The TWO WITCHES *leave their hiding place and close in on* BANCO *from both sides.*

BANCO   What's the meaning of this?

FIRST WITCH   Hail Banco, Macbett's companion.

SECOND WITCH   Hail, General Banco.

BANCO   Who are you? Hideous creatures, what do you want? Lucky for you, you're women—of a kind. Otherwise, I'd have cut your heads off for fooling with me like that.

FIRST WITCH   Now don't get excited, General Banco.

BANCO   How do you know my name?

SECOND WITCH   Hail Banco—who won't be thane of Glamiss.

BANCO   How do you know that title was supposed to be mine? How do you know I won't get it? Has rumor added its murmur to the rustling of the forest? Are wind and storm echoing the news abroad?—Anyway, I can't be thane of Glamiss.

FIRST WITCH   Glamiss is dead. Drowned. The torrent swept him and his horse away.

BANCO   Is this some kind of joke? I'll have your tongues cut out, you old hags.

SECOND WITCH   Duncan is very displeased with you for letting Glamiss escape.

BANCO   How do you know?

FIRST WITCH   He wants to take advantage of this. He's going to give the title, Baron Glamiss, to Macbett. All the estates will revert to the crown.

BANCO   The title alone would have been enough. Why should Duncan wish to deprive me of it? No, Duncan is loyal. He keeps his promises. Why should he give the title to Macbett. Why should he punish me? Why should Macbett have all the favors and all the privileges?

SECOND WITCH   Macbett is your rival. Your successful rival.

BANCO   He is my companion. He is my friend. He is my brother. He is loyal.

The WITCHES *withdraw a little and jump up and down.*

THE TWO WITCHES   He thinks he's loyal. He thinks he's loyal. (*They laugh.*)

BANCO (*drawing his sword*)   Monstrous creatures, I know who you are. You're spies. You're working for the enemies of Duncan, our loyal and beloved sovereign.

He tries to run them through. But they escape and run off, FIRST WITCH *to the left,* SECOND WITCH *to the right.*

FIRST WITCH (*before she disappears*)   Macbett will be king. He'll take Duncan's place.

SECOND WITCH   He'll mount the throne.

BANCO *runs backward and forward brandishing his sword, trying to run them through.*

BANCO   Where are you? Accursed gypsies. Hellish creatures. (*He sheathes his sword and returns to center stage.*) Did I really see them and hear them?

They've changed into the wind and storm. They've changed into the roots of trees. Was it all a dream?

SECOND WITCH'S VOICE Hear me, Banco, hear me. (*The* SECOND WITCH'S VOICE *becomes pleasant and melodious.*) Mark me. You won't be king. But you'll be greater than Macbett. Greater than Macbett. You will found a dynasty which will rule over our country for a thousand years. You will be greater than Macbett—root and father of many kings.

BANCO I don't believe it . . . I don't believe it. (*He takes three or four more swipes, then stops.*) I thought I recognized that voice. Who can it be? Voice, have you a body? Have you a face? Where are you?

VOICE Right beside you. And a long way off. You'll see me again soon. Then you'll know my power and my charm. Till then, Banco.

BANCO I'm shivering. It must be the rain. Or is it fear? Or horror? Or some mysterious longing that this voice arouses in me? Who does it remind me of? Am I already under its spell? (*Change of tone.*) Just ugly old hags, that's all. Spies, intriguers, liars. Father of kings, me? When our beloved sovereign has sons of his own? Macol, who's studying at Carthage, is the natural and legitimate heir to the throne. There's also Donalbain who's just finished a post-graduate degree in business studies at Ragusa. Nonsense, every word of it. I won't give it another thought.

MACBETT'S VOICE Banco! Banco!

BANCO It's Macbett's voice. Macbett! Ah, there you are.

MACBETT'S VOICE Banco!

43

BANCO Macbett! (*He rushes off left, where* MAC-
BETT'S VOICE *was coming from.*)

Pause. The stage is empty.

*Gradually, the light changes. Upstage a sort of enor-
mous moon, very bright, surrounded by big stars. Perhaps the Milky Way, too, like a big bunch of grapes.*

*During the next scene the setting will gradually become
more specific. Little by little we are able to make out
the outline of a castle. In the middle of it, a small
lighted window. It's important that the sets work with
or without the characters.*

*The following sequence can be kept in or cut as re-
quired.*

DUNCAN *crosses silently right to left.*

When he's gone off left, LADY DUNCAN *appears and follows him across. She disappears.*

MACBETT *crosses silently, going the opposite way. An*
OFFICER *crosses silently from right to left.*

BANCO *crosses silently right to left.*

A WOMAN *crosses slowly and silently in the opposite
direction. (I think the woman, at least, should be kept
in.)*

Pause. The stage is empty. BANCO *enters upstage.*

BANCO Well, how about that then? The witch was
  right. Where did she get her information? Does she

have a contact at court? But so quickly. Perhaps she does have supernatural powers after all. Unusual, to say the least. Perhaps she's found a way of harnessing sound waves. Perhaps she's discovered that channel, mentioned in certain myths, that enables you to put the person talking in touch with the person listening. Perhaps she's invented mirrors which reflect distant images as if they were close at hand, as if they were talking to you six feet away. Perhaps she has enchanted glasses that enable her to see for hundreds or thousands of miles. Perhaps she has instruments for amplifying sound and making the ear incredibly sensitive. One of the Archduke's officers has just come to tell me of Glamiss's death and of my being passed over. Did Macbett plot to gain the title? Could my loyal friend and companion be a swindler? Is Duncan so ungrateful that he can disregard my efforts and the risks I've taken, the dangers I've undergone to defend him and keep him from harm? Is there no one I can trust? And shall I then suspect my brother, my faithful dog, the wine I drink, the very air I breathe? No, no. I know Macbett too well to be anything but convinced of his loyalty and his virtue. Duncan's decision is undoubtedly his own; no prompter but his own nature. It shows him in his true colors. But Macbett can't have heard yet. When he does, he'll refuse to have anything to do with it. (*He begins to go off left, then returns center stage.*) They have looked into space, these monstrous daughters of the devil. Can they also look into the future? They told me I should father a line of kings. Strange and incredible. I wish they could tell me more. Perhaps they really do know what will happen. I wish I could see them but I can't . . . But I did.

He goes out left. MACBETT *enters right. Before he comes on we hear him shouting.*

MACBETT   Banco! Banco! (*He comes on. Shouts again, and again.*) Banco! Where can he have got to? They told me he was hereabouts. I wanted to talk to him. A messenger from the Archduke has summoned me to court. The king tells me Glamiss is dead and that I'm to inherit his title, but not his lands. The witches' prophecies are beginning to come true. I tried to tell Duncan that I didn't want him to dispossess Banco in my favor. I tried to tell him that Banco and I were friends and that Banco hadn't done anything to deserve such treatment, that he had served his sovereign loyally. But he wouldn't listen, hear me. If I accept the title, I might lose the friendship of my dear comrade, Banco. If I refuse, I shall incur the king's displeasure. Have I the right to disobey him? I don't disobey when he sends me to war, so I can't very well disobey when he rewards me. That would be contempt. I must explain to Banco. Anyway, Baron Glamiss—it's only a title. There's no money in it, since Duncan's annexed the lands. Yes, I should like to see Banco, but at the same time perhaps I'd rather wait. It's a tricky situation. How did the witches know about it? Will their other predictions come true? It seems impossible. I'd like to know the logic behind it. How do they explain a chain of cause and effect which will set me on the throne? I'd like to hear what they have to say about it—if only to make fun of them. (*He goes out left.*)

Pause. The stage is empty.

The BUTTERFLY HUNTER *comes on left, butterfly net in hand. He is wearing a pale-colored suit and a boater. He has a little black mustache and pince nez. He chases a couple of butterflies and runs off left in pursuit of a third.*

BANCO (*enter right*) Where are those witches? They prophesied Glamiss's death. That's come true. They told me I'd be dispossessed of my rightful title, Baron Glamiss. They told me I should father a long line of kings and princes. Will their prophecy about my descendants come true as well? I'd like to know the logic behind it. How do they explain the chain of cause and effect that will set my posterity on the throne? I'd like to know what they have to say about it—if only to make fun of them. (*He goes out left.*)

Pause. The stage is empty. MACBETT *comes on left. The* FIRST WITCH *has taken up her position stage right unseen by the audience.*

FIRST WITCH (*to* MACBETT. *She speaks in a croaking voice.*) Macbett, you wanted to see me.

Lights up on the WITCH. *She is dressed like a witch, bent double, with a rasping voice. She props herself up on a big stick. She has dirty white unkempt hair.*

MACBETT *jumps. His hand goes instinctively to his sword.*

MACBETT   Cursed hag. You were there all the time.
FIRST WITCH   I came when you called.
MACBETT   On the battlefield I've never been afraid. No enemy has ever frightened me. Bullets have whizzed past my head. I've hacked my way through burning forests. When the flagship was sinking, I wasn't afraid. I jumped into the shark-infested sea and slashed their throats with one hand while swimming with the other. But my hair stands on end when I see this woman's shadow or hear her voice. There's a smell of sulphur in the air. I must use my sword—but as a cross not as a weapon. (*To the* WITCH) You guessed I wanted to speak with you.

The SECOND WITCH *appears behind the* FIRST WITCH *during the following exchange. There needs to be a certain distance—not very great—between them.*

The SECOND WITCH *will need to move slowly from stage left to stage right to arrive in the center of the spot, behind the* FIRST WITCH.

The FIRST WITCH *appears suddenly. A spot comes up on her. The* SECOND WITCH *should emerge more slowly into the light, first of all her head, then her shoulders, then the rest of her body, and her stick. Her shadow enlarged by the lighting will be thrown on the back wall.*

FIRST WITCH   I heard you. I can read your thoughts. I know what you're thinking now and what was going through your mind a few moments ago. You pretended you wanted to see me to make fun of me. You admitted you were afraid. Pull yourself together, general, for Hell's sake. What do you want to know?

MACBETT   Don't you know already?

FIRST WITCH   Some things I know, but some things are beyond my power. Our knowledge is limited, but I can see that, whether you are aware of it or not, your ambition has been kindled. Whatever explanations you may give yourself they are false; they only conceal your true intent.

MACBETT   I want only one thing; to serve my sovereign.

FIRST WITCH   Who are you kidding?

MACBETT   You want to make me believe that I'm other than I am—but you won't succeed.

FIRST WITCH   You're useful to him, otherwise he'd have your head.

MACBETT   My life is his to dispose of.

FIRST WITCH   You're his instrument. You saw how he got you to fight against Glamiss and Candor.

MACBETT   He was right. They were rebels.

FIRST WITCH   He took all Glamiss's lands and half of Candor's.

MACBETT   Everything belongs to the king. Equally the king and all he has belong to us. He is looking after it for us.

FIRST WITCH   And his flunkeys are left to carry the can.

SECOND WITCH   He, he, he, he, he!

MACBETT (*noting the* SECOND WITCH)　Where did she spring from?

FIRST WITCH　He doesn't know how to hold an ax. He doesn't know how to use a scythe.

MACBETT　What do you know about it?

FIRST WITCH　He can't fight himself—he sends others out to do it for him.

SECOND WITCH　He'd be too frightened.

FIRST WITCH　He knows how to steal other people's wives.

SECOND WITCH　Are they part of the public domain too —the King's property?

FIRST WITCH　He demands service from others, although he doesn't know the meaning of the word himself.

MACBETT　I didn't come here to listen to your treasonous lies.

FIRST WITCH　Why did you come and meet me, if that's all we're good for?

MACBETT　I'm beginning to wonder. It was a mistake.

FIRST WITCH　Then bugger off . . .

SECOND WITCH　If you're not interested . . .

FIRST WITCH　You hesitate, I see. So you've decided to stay.

SECOND WITCH　If you'd rather . . .

FIRST WITCH　If it's easier for you . . .

SECOND WITCH　We can disappear.

MACBETT　Stay a little, daughters of Satan. I want to know more.

FIRST WITCH　Be your own master, instead of taking someone else's orders.

SECOND WITCH　Tools he's done with he casts aside. You've outlived your usefulness.

FIRST WITCH   He despises those who are faithful to him.

SECOND WITCH   He thinks they're cowards.

FIRST WITCH   Or fools.

SECOND WITCH   He respects those who stand up to him.

MACBETT   He fights them, too. He beat the rebels Glamiss and Candor.

FIRST WITCH   Macbett beat them, not he.

SECOND WITCH   Glamiss and Candor were his faithful generals before you.

FIRST WITCH   He hated their independence.

SECOND WITCH   He took back what he'd given them.

FIRST WITCH   A fine example of his generosity.

SECOND WITCH   Glamiss and Candor were proud.

FIRST WITCH   And noble. Duncan couldn't stand that.

SECOND WITCH   And courageous.

MACBETT   I won't be another Glamiss. Or another Candor. This time there won't be a Macbett to beat them.

FIRST WITCH   You're beginning to understand.

SECOND WITCH   He, he, he, he!

FIRST WITCH   If you're not careful, he'll have time to find another.

MACBETT   I behaved honorably. I obeyed my sovereign. That's a law of heaven.

SECOND WITCH   It wasn't behaving honorably to fight your peers.

FIRST WITCH   But their death will be useful to you.

SECOND WITCH   He would have used them against you.

FIRST WITCH   Now nothing stands in your way.

SECOND WITCH   You want the throne. Admit it.

MACBETT   No.

FIRST WITCH   It's no good pretending you don't. You're worthy to be king.

SECOND WITCH   You're made for it. It's written in the stars.

MACBETT   You open the slippery slope of temptation before me. Who are you and what do you want? I almost succumbed to your wiles. But I came to my senses in time. Away.

The TWO WITCHES *give ground.*

FIRST WITCH   We're here to open your eyes.

SECOND WITCH   We only want to help you.

FIRST WITCH   It's for your own good.

SECOND WITCH   Justice is all we ask.

FIRST WITCH   True justice.

MACBETT   Stranger and stranger.

SECOND WITCH   He, he, he, he!

MACBETT   Have you really got my interests at heart? Does justice mean so much to you? You old hags, ugly as sin, you shameless old women want to sacrifice your life for my happiness?

SECOND WITCH   Yes, yes, he, he, he, of course.

FIRST WITCH   Because we love you, Macbett. (*Her voice is beginning to alter.*)

SECOND WITCH   It's because she loves you—(*The voice alters.*)—as much as her country, as much as justice, as much as the commonwealth.

FIRST WITCH (*melodious voice*)   It's to help the poor. To bring peace to a country that has known such suffering.

MACBETT   I know that voice.

FIRST WITCH   You know us, Macbett.

MACBETT   For the last time, I order you to tell me who you are or I'll cut your throats for you. (*Taking out sword.*)

SECOND WITCH   Save yourself the trouble.

FIRST WITCH   All in good time, Macbett.

SECOND WITCH   Put back your sword.

> MACBETT *submits.*

And now, Macbett, I want you to watch closely, very closely. Open your eyes. Pin back your ears.

> *The SECOND WITCH circles the FIRST WITCH like a conjuror's assistant. Each time she circles, she jumps two or three times. These jumps develop into a gracious dance as the new aspects of the TWO WITCHES are unveiled. Toward the end the dance becomes slow.*

SECOND WITCH   (*circling the first*)   Quis, quid, ubi . . . quibus auxiliis, cur, quomodo, quando. Felix qui potuit regni cognoscere causas. Fiat lux hic et nunc et fiat voluntas tua. Ad augusta per angusta, ad augusta per angusta. (*The SECOND WITCH takes the FIRST WITCH's stick and throws it away.*) Alter ego surge, alter ego surge.

> *The FIRST WITCH, who was bent double, straightens up.*

> *For this scene—a transformation scene—the FIRST WITCH is center stage, brilliantly lit.*

> *The SECOND WITCH as she circles passes alternately through light and dark areas, depending on*

whether she is downstage or upstage of the FIRST WITCH.

MACBETT, *standing to one side, is in the shade. We are vaguely aware of his startled reactions as the scene progresses.*

The SECOND WITCH *uses her stick like a magic wand. Each time she touches the* FIRST WITCH *with her wand a transformation takes place.*

Obviously the whole scene should be done to music. For the beginning at least some sta~ ~ would be most suitable.

SECOND WITCH (*as before*)   Ante, apud, ad, adversus . . . sus . . .

She touches the FIRST WITCH *with her wand. The* FIRST WITCH *lets fall her old cloak. Undern ath is another old cloak.*

Circum, circa, citra, cis . . .

She touches the FIRST WITCH, *who sheds her old cloak. She is still covered by an ancient shawl that reaches to her feet.*

SECOND WITCH   Cotra, erga, extra, infra . . . (*The* SECOND WITCH *stands up straight.*) Inter, intra, juxta, ob . . . (*As she passes in front of the* FIRST WITCH *she pulls off her glasses.*) Penes, pone, post et praeter . . . (*She pulls off the old shawl. Underneath the shawl a very beautiful dress appears, covered in spangles and glinting stones.*) Prope, propter, per, secundum . . . (*Music more legato and melodious. She pulls off the First Witch's pointed chin.*) Supra, versus, ultra, trans . . .

The FIRST WITCH *sings several notes and trills. The light is sufficiently bright for us to see the First Witch's face and mouth as she sings. She stops singing. The* SECOND WITCH, *as she passes behind the* FIRST, *throws away her stick.*

Video, meliora, deteriora sequor.

MACBETT (*trancelike*) Video meliora, deteriora sequor.

The SECOND WITCH *keeps circling.*

MACBETT *and* FIRST WITCH (*together*) Video meliora, deteriora sequor.

FIRST *and* SECOND WITCHES Video meliora, deteriora sequor.

ALL THREE (*together*) Video meliora, deteriora sequor. Video meliora, deteriora sequor. Video meliora, deteriora sequor.

The SECOND WITCH *removes what's left of the First Witch's mask—i.e., the pointed nose and hairpiece.*

Still circling, she puts a scepter in the First Witch's hands and a crown on her head. Under the lights the FIRST WITCH *appears as if surrounded in a halo of light.*

As she passes behind, the SECOND WITCH *removes her face mask and her old clothes in a single go.*

Now revealed in all her beauty, the FIRST WITCH *becomes* LADY DUNCAN.

The SECOND WITCH *becomes her lady in waiting, equally young and beautiful.*

MACBETT   Oh your Majesty. (*He falls to his knees.*)

The SECOND WITCH, *now Lady Duncan's maid, places a step ladder behind the* FIRST WITCH, *now* LADY DUNCAN, *for her to climb.*

If this can't be managed, LADY DUNCAN *walks backward, slowly and majestically, stage right, where there is a ladder which she proceeds to mount.*

MACBETT *gets up and once more throws himself at Lady Duncan's feet.*

MACBETT   Oh mirabile visu! Oh madam!

In one movement, the LADY IN WAITING *tears off Lady Duncan's sumptuous dress.* LADY DUNCAN *stands revealed in a sparkling bikini, a black-and-red cape on her back and holding a scepter in one hand and in the other a dagger which the* LADY IN WAITING *has given her.*

LADY IN WAITING (*pointing to* LADY DUNCAN)   In naturalibus.

MACBETT   Let me be your slave.

LADY DUNCAN (*to* MACBETT, *holding out the dagger to him*)   I'll be yours if you wish. Would you like that? Here is the instrument of your ambition and our rise to power. (*Seductively.*) Take it if that's what you want, if you want me. But act boldly. Hell helps those who help themselves. Look into yourself. You can feel your desire for me growing, your hidden ambition coming into the open, inflaming you. You'll take his place at my side. I'll be your mistress. You'll be my sovereign. An indelible bloodstain will mark this blade—a souvenir of your success and a spur to greater things which we shall accomplish with the same glory. (*She raises him up.*)

MACBETT   Madam, sire, or rather siren . . .

LADY DUNCAN   Still hesitating, Macbett?

LADY IN WAITING (*to* LADY DUNCAN)   Make up his mind for him.

LADY DUNCAN   Make up your mind.

MACBETT   Madam, I have certain scruples . . . can't we just . . .

LADY DUNCAN   I know you're brave. But even brave men have their weaknesses and moments of cowardice. Above all they suffer from guilt—and that's mortal. Pull yourself together. You were never afraid to kill when someone else was giving the orders. If fear now weighs you down, unburden yourself to me. I'll reassure you, promise you that no man of woman born will be able to conquer you. No other army will defeat your army till the forest arms itself to march against you.

LADY IN WAITING   Which is practically impossible. (*To* MACBETT) Remember we want only to save our country. The two of you will build a better society, a brave new world.

The stage grows gradually darker.

MACBETT *rolls at Lady Duncan's feet. All that can be seen is Lady Duncan's glistening body. We hear the voice of the* LADY IN WAITING.

LADY IN WAITING   Omnia vincit amor.

Blackout.

A room in the palace.

In front of the palace, BANCO *and an* OFFICER.

OFFICER His Highness is tired. He can't see you now.

BANCO Does he know what I've come for?

OFFICER I explained everything, but he says it's a *fait accompli*. He's given Glamiss's title to Macbett and he can't very well take it back again. Besides, it's only his word.

BANCO But still . . .

OFFICER That's the way it is.

BANCO Does he know Glamiss is dead, drowned?

OFFICER I told him, but he'd already heard. Lady Duncan knew of it through her Lady in Waiting.

BANCO There's no reason why he shouldn't give me my promised reward. The title or the lands, if not both.

OFFICER What do you want me to do? I've done my best?

BANCO It's impossible. He can't do this to me.

Enter DUNCAN *stage right.*

DUNCAN (*to* BANCO)   What's all the fuss about?

BANCO   My lord—

DUNCAN   I don't like being disturbed. What do you want?

BANCO   Didn't you tell me, that when Glamiss had been taken, dead or alive, you'd give me my reward?

DUNCAN   Where is he? Dead or alive I don't see him.

BANCO   You know very well he's drowned.

DUNCAN   That's hearsay. Bring me his body.

BANCO   His bloated corpse has been swept out to sea.

DUNCAN   Well go and look for it. Take a boat.

BANCO   The sharks have eaten it.

DUNCAN   Take a knife and cut through the shark's belly.

BANCO   Several sharks.

DUNCAN   Cut through all their bellies then.

BANCO   I risked my life defending you against the rebels.

DUNCAN   You've come out of it alive, haven't you?

BANCO   I killed all your enemies.

DUNCAN   You had that pleasure.

BANCO   I could've done without it.

DUNCAN   But you didn't

BANCO   My lord—

DUNCAN   Not another word. Where is Glamiss's body? Show me the *corpus delicti*.

BANCO   Glamiss's death is common knowledge. You've given his title to Macbett.

DUNCAN   Are you demanding an explanation?

BANCO   It's not fair.

DUNCAN   I'll be the judge of that. We'll find other rebel barons to dispossess. There's bound to be something for you in the future.

BANCO   I'm afraid I think you're lying.

DUNCAN   How dare you insult me?

BANCO   But . . . but . . .

DUNCAN   Show this gentleman the door.

The OFFICER *appears to be on the point of launching himself violently at* BANCO. *He shouts.*

OFFICER   Out!

DUNCAN   No need for rough stuff. Banco is a good friend of ours. His nerves are a little on edge, that's all. He'll get over it. He'll get his opportunity.

BANCO (*going out*)   What a bloody sauce . . .

DUNCAN (*to the* OFFICER)   I don't know what got into me. I should have made him Baron. But he wanted the money, too, which should rightfully have reverted to me. Well, that's the way it is. But if he gets dangerous, we shall have to be careful—very careful.

OFFICER (*putting his hand on his sword*)   I understand, my lord.

DUNCAN   No, no, not so fast. Not immediately. Later. If he becomes dangerous. Would you like his title and half his lands?

OFFICER (*energetically*)   Yes, my lord. Whatever you say, my lord.

DUNCAN   You're a thrusting little codger, aren't you? I suppose you'd like me to confiscate Macbett's title and fortune and give you a bit of that as well?

OFFICER (*as before*)   Yes, my lord. Whatever you say, my lord.

DUNCAN   Macbett is also becoming dangerous. Very dangerous. Perhaps he'd like to replace me on the throne. That sort of person needs to be watched.

6 1

Hoodlums, that's what they are, gangsters. All they think about is money, power, luxury. I wouldn't be surprised if Macbett also had an eye on my wife. Not to mention my courtesans. How about you? Would you like me to lend you my wife?

OFFICER (*protesting energetically*) Oh no, my lord.

DUNCAN Don't you fancy her?

OFFICER She is very beautiful, my lord. But honor, your honor comes first.

DUNCAN That's a good chap. Thanks. I'll see that you're rewarded.

OFFICER Whatever you say, my lord.

DUNCAN I'm surrounded by grasping enemies and fickle friends. Nobody is unselfish. You'd think the prosperity of the kingdom and my personal well-being would satisfy them. They've got no ideals. None at all. We shall be on our guard.

Fanfares and music. Something old fashioned and formal.

A room in the Archduke's Palace. Just a few items, one or two chairs and a different backcloth, will do to establish the locality. Whatever can be set up in a blackout lasting not more than thirty seconds.

Music. DUNCAN *enters right, followed by* LADY DUNCAN. *He is agitated and she has difficulty keeping up with him.*

DUNCAN *comes to a sudden halt center stage. He turns to* LADY DUNCAN.

DUNCAN   No. madam, I won't allow it.

LADY DUNCAN   So much the worse for you.

DUNCAN   I said, I won't allow it.

LADY DUNCAN   Why not? Why ever not?

DUNCAN   Let me speak frankly, with my customary candor.

LADY DUNCAN   Frankly or not it all boils down to the same thing.

DUNCAN   What do I care?

LADY DUNCAN   You said I could. It's no good denying it.

DUNCAN   I shall if I want. I said perhaps.

LADY DUNCAN   What about me? What am I supposed to say?

DUNCAN   Whatever comes into your head.

LADY DUNCAN   I never say whatever comes into my head.

DUNCAN   If it isn't in your head how can you say it?

LADY DUNCAN   First one thing, then another. Tomorrow it'll be something else again.

DUNCAN   I can't help that.

LADY DUNCAN   Neither can I.

DUNCAN   Stop contradicting.

LADY DUNCAN   You're always putting things off.

DUNCAN   You've only yourself to blame.

LADY DUNCAN   You're such an old fuss-pot.

DUNCAN   Madam, madam, madam!

LADY DUNCAN   You're being very stubborn. Men are so self-centered.

DUNCAN   Let's get back to the subject in hand.

LADY DUNCAN   It's no good your getting cross, it only makes me cross as well. The most important thing is done. If you were more objective about it . . . but you aren't. So, let's leave it. It's all your fault.

DUNCAN   Hold your tongue, madam. He who laughs last, laughs longest.

LADY DUNCAN   Your obsessions, your *idées fixes*.

DUNCAN   That'll do.

LADY DUNCAN   So you still refuse . . .

DUNCAN   You'll regret it.

LADY DUNCAN   You can't make an omelette without breaking eggs.

DUNCAN   You'll pay dearly.

LADY DUNCAN   Are you threatening me?

DUNCAN   From top to toe.

LADY DUNCAN   Another threat!

DUNCAN   One day you'll go too far.

LADY DUNCAN   And another!

DUNCAN   I won't have it. No, absolutely not. You just wait. The shoe will be on the other foot. I'll tell him. You see if I don't. I'll rub his nose in it.

DUNCAN *goes out quickly, followed by* LADY DUNCAN.

LADY DUNCAN   I'll forestall you, Duncan. By the time you find out it'll be too late.

DUNCAN, *still agitated, has gone out left after his last speech.* LADY DUNCAN *follows him out, almost at a run.*

The scene between the two of them should be played as a violent quarrel.

MACBETT *and* BANCO *enter right.* MACBETT *looks worried. He has a serious air about him.*

MACBETT   No, seriously. I thought Lady Duncan was a shallow woman. I was wrong. She is capable of deep feeling. She is so vivacious, energetic. She really is. And intellectual. She has some very profound views on the future of mankind: though she's by no means a utopian dreamer.

BANCO   It's possible. I believe you. It's difficult to get to know people, but once they've opened their hearts to you . . . (*Pointing to Macbett's belt.*) That's a handsome dagger that you've got there.

MACBETT   A gift from her. Anyway, I'm glad to have had a chance to talk with you at long last after all this chasing about like a dog after its own tail or the devil chasing his shadow.

BANCO   You can say that again.

MACBETT   She's unhappily married. Duncan is a brute. He maltreats her. It's very trying. She's very delicate, you know. And he's peevish and broody. Lady Duncan is like a child—she likes to sport and amuse herself, play tennis, make love. Of course, it's none of my business, really.

BANCO   Of course.

MACBETT   Far be it from me to speak ill of the king or want to run him down.

BANCO   Perish the thought.

MACBETT   The Archduke is a very good man, loyal and . . . generous. You know how fond I am of him.

BANCO   Me, too.

MACBETT   All in all he's a perfect monarch.

BANCO   Almost perfect.

MACBETT   Obviously, as far as perfection is possible in this world. It's a perfection that doesn't exclude certain imperfections.

BANCO   An imperfect perfection. But perfection all the same.

MACBETT   Personally, I've got nothing against him—though my own opinion doesn't enter into it. He has the good of the country at heart. Yes, he's a good king. Though he should be more appreciative of his impartial advisers—like you, for example.

BANCO   Or you.

MACBETT   Like you or me.

BANCO   Quite.

MACBETT   He's a bit autocratic.

BANCO   Very autocratic.

MACBETT   A real autocrat! Nowadays autocracy isn't always the best way to govern. That's what Lady Duncan thinks anyway. She's very charming, you know, and has a lot of interesting ideas, two qualities that aren't often found together.

BANCO   Not often, no.

MACBETT   She could give him some good advice, interesting advice, get him to see . . . to understand certain principles of government which, in an impartial way, she would share with us. We ourselves, of course, being quite impartial.

BANCO   All the same we've got to live, earn our daily bread.

MACBETT   Duncan understands that.

BANCO   Yes, he's shown himself very understanding so far as you're concerned. He's showered you with blessings.

MACBETT   I didn't ask him to. He paid, he paid well, well more or less—he didn't pay too badly for the services I rendered him—which it was my duty to render, since he is my feudal overlord.

BANCO   He didn't pay me at all! As you know. He took Glamiss's lands for himself and gave you the title.

MACBETT   I don't know what you're referring to. Duncan do a thing like that? Never—well, hardly ever—well, not very often. He has his lapses. I didn't intrigue for it, I promise.

BANCO   I never said you did. I know it's not your fault.

MACBETT   It's not my fault. Listen: perhaps we can do something for you. We—Lady Duncan and I that is—we could advise him. We could, for example, advise him to take you on as his adviser.

BANCO   Lady Duncan knows about this, does she?

MACBETT   She's very concerned about you. She's very upset by the king's thoughtlessness. She wants to make it up to you. She's already put in a word for you with the Archduke, you know. I suggested it to her, and she agreed. We've both intervened on your behalf.

BANCO   Why keep on if your attempts have been unsuccessful?

MACBETT   We'll use other arguments. More cogent ones. Then perhaps he'll understand. If not . . . we'll try again. With even stronger arguments.

BANCO   Duncan is stubborn.

MACBETT   Very stubborn. Stubborn . . . (*He looks left and right.*) . . . as stubborn as a mule. Still, even the stubbornest mule can be made to budge.

BANCO   Made to, yes.

MACBETT   Fair enough, he's given me the estates—but he's reserved the right to hunt on my lands. Apparently, it's for "state expenses."

BANCO   So he says . . .

MACBETT   He *is* the state.

BANCO   My estates are still the same as ever and he takes from me ten thousand chickens a year and their eggs.

MACBETT   You should complain.

BANCO   I fought for him at the head of my own personal army. Now he wants to merge it with his army. He wants to turn my own men against me.

MACBETT   And me.

BANCO   My ancestors would turn over in their graves . . .

MACBETT   So would mine! And there's all his cronies and parasites.

BANCO   Who fat themselves on the sweat of our brow.

MACBETT   And our chickens.

BANCO   And our sheep.

MACBETT   And our pigs.

BANCO   The swine.

MACBETT   And our bread.

BANCO   The blood we've shed for him.

MACBETT   The dangers we've undergone.

BANCO   Ten thousand chickens, ten thousand horses, ten thousand recruits. What does he do with them? He can't eat them all. The rest just goes bad.

MACBETT   And a thousand young girls.

BANCO   We know what he does with them.

MACBETT   He owes us everything.

BANCO   More than he can pay.

MACBETT   Not to mention the rest.

BANCO   My honor.

MACBETT   My glory.

BANCO   Our ancestral rights.

MACBETT   My property.

BANCO   The right to make more and more money.

MACBETT   Self-rule.

BANCO   To run our own affairs.

MACBETT   We must drive him out.

BANCO   Lock, stock and barrel. Down with Duncan.

MACBETT   Down with Duncan!

BANCO   We must overthrow him.

MACBETT   I was going to suggest . . . we should divide the kingdom. We'll each have our share and I'll take the throne. I'll be king and you can be my chamberlain.

BANCO   Your second-in-command.

MACBETT   Well third, actually. It's a difficult task we've set ourselves and we need all the help we can get. There is a third in this conspiracy—Lady Duncan.

BANCO   Well, well. That's a piece of luck.

MACBETT   She's indispensable.

LADY DUNCAN *enters upstage.*

BANCO   Madam! What a surprise.

MACBETT (*to* BANCO)   We're engaged.

BANCO   The future Lady Macbett. Well, well. (*Looking from one to the other.*) Heartiest congratulations. (*He kisses Lady Duncan's hand.*)

LADY DUNCAN   To the death!

They all three draw their daggers and cross them at arm's length.

Let's swear to kill the tyrant!

MACBETT   The usurper.

BANCO   Down with the dictator!

LADY DUNCAN   The despot.

MACBETT   He's a miscreant.

BANCO   An ogre.

LADY DUNCAN   An ass.

MACBETT   A goose.

BANCO   A louse.

LADY DUNCAN   Let's swear to exterminate him.

ALL THREE (*together*)   We swear to exterminate him.

Fanfares. The conspirators go out quickly left.

The ARCHDUKE *comes on right. In this scene, at least at the beginning,* DUNCAN *has real majesty.*

Enter the OFFICER *upstage.*

OFFICER   My lord, it's the first day of the month, the day when the scrofulous, the tubercular, the consumptive, and the hysterical come for you to cure their maladies by your heavenly gift.

A MONK *comes on left.*

MONK   Greetings, my lord.

DUNCAN   Greetings, father.

MONK   God be with you.

DUNCAN   And with you.

MONK   May the lord preserve you. (*He blesses the Archduke, who bows his head.*)

The OFFICER, *carrying the king's purple robe, the crown, and the royal scepter, goes over to the* MONK.

The MONK *blesses the crown and takes it from the* OFFICER. *He goes over to* DUNCAN, *who kneels down, and puts it on his head.*

MONK   In the name of Almighty God, I confirm you in your sovereign power.

DUNCAN   May the lord make me worthy.

The OFFICER *gives the purple cloak to the* MONK *who puts it around Duncan's shoulders.*

MONK   May the Lord bless you and keep you, and may no harm come to you so long as you wear this cloak.

A SERVANT *comes on right carrying the ciborium for communion. He gives it to the* MONK *who offers* DUNCAN *the Host.*

DUNCAN   Domine non sum dignus.

MONK   Corpus Christi.

DUNCAN   Amen.

The MONK *gives the ciborium back to the* SERVANT, *who goes out.*

The OFFICER *hands the* MONK *the scepter.*

MONK   I renew the gift of healing which the Lord God transmits through me, his unworthy servant. May the Lord purge our souls as he heals the sickness of our feeble bodies. May He cure us of jealousy, pride, luxury, our base striving after power, and may He open our eyes to the vanity of worldly goods.

DUNCAN   Hear us, O Lord.

OFFICER (*kneeling*)   Hear us, O Lord.

MONK   Hear us, O Lord. May hatred and anger waft away like smoke in the wind. Grant that man may prevail against nature, where suffering and destruction reign. May love and peace be freed from their chains, may all destructive forces be chained up that joy may shine forth in heavenly light. May that light flood us that we may bathe ourselves in it. Amen.

DUNCAN *and* OFFICER   Amen.

MONK   Take your scepter with my blessing. With it you are to touch the sick.

> DUNCAN *and the* OFFICER *get up. The* MONK *kneels before* DUNCAN *who mounts the throne and sits. The* OFFICER *stands on Duncan's left. This scene should be played with solemnity.*

DUNCAN   Bring in the patients.

> *The* MONK *rises and goes and stands on Duncan's right.*

> *The* FIRST SICK MAN *comes in upstage left. He is bent double and walks with difficulty. He is wearing a cape with a hood. His face is a ravaged mask —like a leper's.*

Come here. A little nearer. Don't be afraid.

> *The* SICK MAN *approaches and kneels on one of the bottom steps of the throne. He has his back to the audience.*

FIRST SICK MAN   Have pity on me, my lord. I've come
a long way. On the other side of the ocean, there is a
continent and beyond that continent, there are seven
countries. And beyond those seven countries there's
another sea, and beyond that sea there are mountains. I live on the other side of those mountains in a
damp and sunless valley. The damp has eaten away
my bones. I'm covered in scrofula, in tumors and
pustules which break out everywhere. My body is a
running sore. I stink. My wife and children can't
bear me to come near them. Save me, lord. Cure me.
DUNCAN   I shall cure you. Believe in me and hope. (*He
touches the Sick Man's head with his scepter.*) By
the grace of our Lord Jesus Christ, by the gift of the
power vested in me this day, I absolve you of the sin
which has stained your soul and body. May your
soul be as pure as clear water, as the sky on the first
day of creation.

> The FIRST SICK MAN *stands up and turns toward
> the audience. He draws himself up to his full
> height, drops his stick and lifts his hands to
> heaven.*
>
> *His face is clear and smiling. He shouts for joy
> and runs out left.*
>
> The SECOND SICK MAN *enters right and approaches
> the throne.*

DUNCAN   What is your trouble?
SECOND SICK MAN   My lord, I'm unable to live and I
can't die. I can't sit down, I can't lie down, I can't

stand still, and I can't run. I burn and itch from the top of my head to the soles of my feet. I can't bear to be indoors or on the street. For me, the universe is a prison. It pains me to look at the world. I can't bear the light nor sit in the shade. Other people fill me with horror, yet I can't bear to be alone. My eyes wander restlessly over trees, sheep, dogs, grass, stars, stones. I have never had a single happy moment. I should like to be able to cry, my lord, and to know joy. (*During this speech, he has come up to the throne and climbed the steps.*)

DUNCAN   Forget you exist. Remember that you are.

Pause.

Seen from behind, one can read in the twitching of the Sick Man's shoulders that it's impossible for him to comply.

I order you. Obey.

The SECOND SICK MAN, *who was twisted in agony, relaxes his back and shoulders and appears to be calming down. He gets up slowly, holds out his arms and turns around. The audience can see the contorted face relax and light up.*

He walks off left, jauntily, almost dancing.

OFFICER   Next!

A THIRD SICK MAN *approaches* DUNCAN, *who cures him in the same way. Then in quick succession a Fourth, Fifth, Sixth . . . Tenth, Eleventh come on stage right and go out left after having been touched by Duncan's scepter.*

Before each entrance, the OFFICER *shouts "Next!"*

Some of the Patients are on crutches or in wheelchairs.

All this should be properly controlled and toward the end should be accompanied by music which gradually gets faster and faster.

While this is going on, the MONK *has slowly dropped away till he is sitting rather than kneeling on the floor. He looks poised.*

After the Eleventh SICK MAN, *the tempo becomes slower and the music fades into the distance.*

Two last patients come in, one from the left, the other from the right. They are wearing long capes with hoods that come down over their faces. The OFFICER *who shouted "Next" fails to notice the last patient, who creeps up behind him.*

Suddenly the music cuts out. At the same moment, the MONK *throws back his hood or takes off his mask, and we see that it's* BANCO *in disguise. He pulls out a long dagger.*

DUNCAN (*to* BANCO) You?

At the same moment, LADY DUNCAN *throws off her disguise and stabs the* OFFICER *in the back. He falls.*

DUNCAN (*to* LADY DUNCAN) You, madam?

*The other beggar—*MACBETT*—also pulls out a dagger.*

DUNCAN Murderers!
BANCO (*to* DUNCAN) Murderer!
MACBETT (*to* DUNCAN) Murderer!

DUNCAN dodges BANCO *and comes face to face with* MACBETT. *He tries to go out left but his escape is cut off by* LADY DUNCAN, *who holds out her arms to stop him. She has a dagger in one hand.*

LADY DUNCAN (*to* DUNCAN) Murderer!
DUNCAN (*to* LADY DUNCAN) Murderess! (*He runs left, meets* MACBETT.)
MACBETT Murderer!
DUNCAN Murderer! (*He runs right.* BANCO *cuts him off.*)
BANCO (*to* DUNCAN) Murderer!
DUNCAN (*to* BANCO) Murderer!

DUNCAN backs toward the throne. The three others close in on him, slowly drawing their circle tighter.

As DUNCAN *mounts the first step,* LADY DUNCAN *snatches off his cloak.* DUNCAN *backs up the steps trying to cover his body with his arms. Without his cloak he feels naked and exposed.*

He doesn't get very far, however, for the others are after him. His scepter falls one way, his crown the other. MACBETT *pulls at him and brings him down.*

DUNCAN   Murderers!

He rolls on the ground. BANCO *strikes the first blow, shouting.*

BANCO   Murderer!
MACBETT (*stabbing him a second time*)   Murderer!
LADY DUNCAN (*stabbing him a third time*)   Murderer!

The three of them get up and stand over him.

DUNCAN   Murderers! (*Quieter.*) Murderers! (*Feebly.*) Murderers!

The three conspirators draw apart. LADY DUNCAN *stays by the body, looking down.*

LADY DUNCAN   He was my husband, after all. Now that he's dead, he looks just like my father. I couldn't stand my father.

Blackout.

A room in the palace. In the distance we can hear the crowd shouting, "Long live Macbett! Long live his bride! Long live Macbett! Long live his bride!"

Two SERVANTS *enter upstage, one from one side, one from the other. They meet downstage center. They can be played by two men, or a man and a woman, possibly even two women.*

SERVANTS (*looking at each other*)   They're coming.

> *They go and hide upstage. Enter left Duncan's widow, the future* LADY MACBETT, *followed by* MACBETT. *They have not as yet acquired the regal attributes.*
>
> *The cheering and shouts of "Long live Macbett and his bride" are louder.*
>
> *They go to the exit stage left.*

LADY DUNCAN   Thank you for bringing me to my apartments. I'm going to lie down. I'm quite tired after my exertions.

MACBETT Yes, you could do with a rest. I'll come and pick you up at ten o'clock for the marriage ceremony. The coronation is at midday. In the afternoon, at five o'clock, there will be a banquet—our wedding feast.

LADY DUNCAN (*giving her hand to* MACBETT *to be kissed*) Till tomorrow then, Macbett.

She goes out. MACBETT *crosses to go out right. The sound of scattered cheering.*

The two SERVANTS *who had hidden reappear and come downstage.*

FIRST SERVANT Everything is ready for the wedding ceremony and the breakfast afterward.

SECOND SERVANT Wines from Italy and Samoa.

FIRST SERVANT Bottles of beer coming by the dozen.

SECOND SERVANT And gin.

FIRST SERVANT Oxen.

SECOND SERVANT Herds of deer.

FIRST SERVANT Roebuck to be barbecued.

SECOND SERVANT They've come from France, from the Ardennes.

FIRST SERVANT Fishermen have risked their lives to provide sharks. They'll eat the fins.

SECOND SERVANT They killed a whale for oil to dress the salad.

FIRST SERVANT There'll be Pernod from Marseille.

SECOND SERVANT Vodka from the Urals.

FIRST SERVANT A giant omelette containing a hundred and thirty thousand eggs.

SECOND SERVANT Chinese pancakes.

FIRST SERVANT Spanish melons from Africa.

SECOND SERVANT   There's never been anything like it.

FIRST SERVANT   Viennese pastries.

SECOND SERVANT   Wine will flow like water in the streets.

FIRST SERVANT   To the sound of a dozen gypsy orchestras.

SECOND SERVANT   Better than Christmas.

FIRST SERVANT   A thousand times better.

SECOND SERVANT   Everyone in the country will get two hundred and forty-seven black sausages.

FIRST SERVANT   And a ton of mustard.

SECOND SERVANT   Frankfurters.

FIRST SERVANT   And sauerkraut.

SECOND SERVANT   And more beer.

FIRST SERVANT   And more wine.

SECOND SERVANT   And more gin.

FIRST SERVANT   I'm drunk already, just thinking about it.

SECOND SERVANT   Just thinking about it I can feel my belly bursting.

FIRST SERVANT   My liver swelling. (*They throw their arms around each other's necks and stagger out drunkenly, shouting "Long live Macbett and his bride."*)

BANCO *enters right. He crosses to stage center and stops, facing the audience. He appears to reflect for a moment.* MACBETT *appears upstage left.*

MACBETT   Ah, it's Banco. What's he doing here all by himself? I'll hide and overhear him. (*He pretends to pull invisible curtains.*)

BANCO   So Macbett is to be king; Baron Candor, Baron

Glamiss, then king—as from tomorrow. One by one
the witches' predictions have come true. One thing
they didn't mention was the murder of Duncan, in
which I had a hand. But how would Macbett have
come to power unless Duncan had died or abdicated
in his favor—which is constitutionally impossible?
You have to take the throne by force. Another thing
they didn't mention was that Lady Duncan would be
Lady Macbett. So Macbett gets everything—while I
get nothing. What an extraordinarily successful
career—wealth, fame, power, a wife. He's got everything a man could possibly want. I struck down Duncan because I had a grudge against him. But what
good has it done me? True, Macbett has given me his
word. He said I could be chamberlain. But will he
keep his promise? I doubt it. Didn't he promise to be
faithful to Duncan—and then kill him? People will
say I did the same. I can't say I didn't. I can't get it
out of my mind. I'm sorry now—and I haven't any of
Macbett's advantages, his success, his fame, to stifle
my remorse. The witches told me I shouldn't be
archduke or king, but they said I should father a
whole line of kings, princes, presidents, and dicta-
tors. That's some consolation. They said it would
happen, yes, they said it would happen. They've
proved conclusively that they can see into the future.
Before I met them I had no desire, no ambition beyond that of serving my king. Now I'm consumed
with envy and jealousy. They've taken the lid off my
ambition and here I am carried away by a force I
can't control—grasping, avid, insatiable. I shall
father dozens of kings. That's something. But yet
I have no sons or daughters. And I'm not married.

Whom shall I marry? The Lady in Waiting is rather sexy. I'll ask her to marry me. She's a bit spooky but so much the better. She'll be able to see danger coming and we can take steps to avoid it. Once I'm married, once I've started a family, once I'm chamberlain, I'll curtail Macbett's powers. I'll be his *éminence gris*. Who knows, perhaps the witches will reconsider their predictions. Perhaps I will reign in my own lifetime after all. (*He goes out right.*)

MACBETT   I heard every word, the traitor! So that's all the thanks I get for promising to make him chamberlain. I didn't know my wife and her maid had told him that he'd be father to a line of kings. Funny she never mentioned it. It's disturbing to think she kept it from me. Who are they trying to fool, me or Banco? Why? Banco father to a line of kings. Have I killed Duncan to put Banco's issue on the throne? It's all a sinister plot. Well, we'll soon see about that. We'll soon see if my initiative can foil the snares of destiny the devil has set for me. Let's destroy his issue at the fountainhead—that is, Banco himself. (*He crosses right and calls.*) Banco! Banco!

BANCO'S VOICE   Coming, Macbett. Coming. (BANCO *comes on.*) What do you want?

MACBETT   Coward, so that is how you repay me for all the favors I was going to grant you. (*He stabs* BANCO *in the heart.*)

BANCO (*falling*)   Oh my God! Have mercy.

MACBETT   Where are all those kings now? They're going to rot with you and in you, nipped in the bud. (*He goes.*)

Blackout.

Lights up.

Shouts of "Long live Macbett! Long live Lady Macbett! Long live our beloved king! Long live the bride!"

MACBETT *and* LADY MACBETT *come on right. They are in robes of state. They wear crowns and purple robes.*

MACBETT *is carrying his scepter. Sound of bells ringing and the enthusiastic cheering of the crowd.* MACBETT *and* LADY MACBETT *stop center stage with their backs to the audience and wave left and right to the crowd.*

Noise of the crowd: "Hurrah! Long live the Archduke! Long live the Archduchess!"

MACBETT *and* LADY MACBETT *turn and salute the audience, waving and blowing kisses. They turn and face each other.*

MACBETT   We'll discuss it later.
LADY MACBETT   I can explain everything, dear.
MACBETT   Well, I've canceled your prediction. I've nipped it in the bud. You've no longer got the upper

hand. I discovered your little arrangements and took steps accordingly.

LADY MACBETT   I didn't mean to hide anything from you, love. As I said, I can explain everything. But not in public.

MACBETT   We'll discuss it later.

> MACBETT *takes her hand and they go out right, smiling at the crowd. The cheering continues.*
>
> *Pause. The stage is empty.* LADY MACBETT *comes on with her* LADY IN WAITING. *She is in the same costume as in the previous scene.*

LADY IN WAITING   It suits you, being a bride. The crowd cheering. The way you held yourself. Such grace. Such majesty. He cut a fine figure, too. He's looking much younger. You made a lovely couple.

LADY MACBETT   He's gone to sleep. He had a few too many after the ceremony. And there's still the wedding feast to come. Let's make the most of it. Hurry up.

LADY IN WAITING   Yes, ma'am. (*She collects a case from offstage right.*)

LADY MACBETT   Away with this sacred and anointed crown. (*She throws the crown away. She takes off the necklace with a cross on it which she had been wearing.*) This cross has been burning me. I've got a wound, here on my chest. But I've doused it with curses.

> *Meanwhile the* LADY IN WAITING *has been opening the case and taking out her witch's costume. She proceeds to dress* LADY MACBETT *in it.*

The cross symbolizes the struggle of two forces, heaven and hell. Which will prove the stronger? Within this small compass a universal warfare is condensed. Help me. Undo my white dress. Quickly, take it off. It's burning me as well. And I spit out the Host which fortunately stuck in my throat. Give me the flask of spiced and magic vodka. Alcohol 90 proof is like mineral water to me. Twice I nearly fainted when they held up the icons for me to touch. But I carried it off. I even kissed one of them. Pouah, it was disgusting.

> *During all this, the* LADY IN WAITING *is undressing her.*

Hurry up. I hear something.
LADY IN WAITING   Yes, ma'am. I'm doing my best.
LADY MACBETT   Hurry, hurry, hurry. Give me my rags, my smelly old dress. My apron covered in vomit. My muddy boots. Take this wig off. Where's my dirty gray hair? Give me my chin. Here, take these teeth. My pointed nose, and my stick tipped with poisoned steel.

> *The* LADY IN WAITING *picks up one of the sticks left by the pilgrims.*

> *As* LADY MACBETT *issues her orders, "Unhook my white dress!" etc., the* LADY IN WAITING *carries them out.*

> *As indicated in the text, she puts on her smelly old dress, her apron covered in vomit, her dirty*

gray hair, takes out her teeth, shows the plate to audience, puts on her pointed nose, etc.

FIRST WITCH   Hurry! Faster!
SECOND WITCH   I am hurrying, my dear.
FIRST WITCH   They are waiting for us.

The SECOND WITCH *produces a long shawl from the case and puts it around her shoulders, at the same time pulling on a dirty gray wig.*

The two WITCHES *are bent double and sniggering.*

I feel much more at home, dressed like this.
SECOND WITCH   He, he, he, he!

She shuts the case. They both sit astride it.

FIRST WITCH   Well, that's that, then.
SECOND WITCH   A job well done.
FIRST WITCH   We've mixed it nicely.
SECOND WITCH   He, he, he, he. Macbett won't be able to get out of it now.
FIRST WITCH   The boss will be pleased.
SECOND WITCH   We'll tell him all about it.
FIRST WITCH   He'll be waiting to send us on another mission.
SECOND WITCH   Let's skedaddle. Suitcase, fly!
FIRST WITCH   Fly! Fly! Fly!

The FIRST WITCH, *who is sitting in front of the case, mimes a steering wheel. It's a very noisy engine. The* SECOND WITCH *spreads her arms, like wings.*

MACBETT

Blackout. Spotlight on the case which appears to be flying.

The main hall of the palace. Upstage, the throne. Downstage and a little to the left, a table with stools. Four GUESTS *are already seated.*

Four or five life-size dolls represent the other GUESTS. *Upstage, other tables and other* GUESTS *projected onto the back wall on either side of the throne.*

MACBETT *comes on left.*

MACBETT   Don't get up, my friends.

FIRST GUEST   Long live the Archduke!

SECOND GUEST   Long live our sovereign!

THIRD GUEST   Long live Macbett!

FOURTH GUEST   Long live our guide! Our great captain! Our Macbett!

MACBETT   Thank you, friends.

FIRST GUEST   Glory and honor and health to our beloved sovereign, Lady Macbett!

FOURTH GUEST   Her beauty and her grace make her worthy of your highness. May you live and prosper. May the state flourish under your wise and powerful rule, guided and helped by your lady wife.

MACBETT   Accept my thanks for both. She should have been here by now.

SECOND GUEST   Her Highness is never late normally.

MACBETT   I left her only a few minutes ago. She and her maid were right behind me.

THIRD GUEST   Has she taken ill? I'm a doctor.

MACBETT   She's gone to her room to put on some lipstick, a dab of powder, and a new necklace. In the meanwhile, don't stop drinking. I'll come and join you.

A SERVANT *comes on.*

There's not enough wine. More wine there!

SERVANT   I'll go and get some, my lord.

MACBETT   Your health, my friends. How happy I am to be with you. I feel surrounded by the warmth of your affection. If you knew how much I need your friendship—as much as a plant needs water or a man wine. I find it consoling, soothing, reassuring, having you around me. Ah, if only you knew . . . But I mustn't let myself go. It's not the moment for confessions. You set out to do something and end up doing something quite different, which you didn't intend at all. History is full of tricks like that. Everything slips through your fingers. We unleash forces that we cannot control and which end up by turning against us. Everything turns out the opposite of what you wanted. Man doesn't rule events, events rule him. I was happy when I was serving Duncan faithfully. I hadn't a care in the world.

The SERVANT *comes in.* MACBETT *turns toward him.*

Quickly, we're dying of thirst. (*Looking at a portrait —it could just as easily be an empty frame.*) Who put Duncan's picture in my place? Is this someone's idea of a joke?

SERVANT I don't know, my lord. I didn't see anything, my lord.

MACBETT How dare you. (*He takes the* SERVANT *by the throat, then lets him go again. He goes to unhook the portrait—which could equally well be an empty frame or invisible.*)

FIRST GUEST But that's your picture, my lord.

SECOND GUEST They put your picture where Duncan's was, not vice versa.

MACBETT It does look like him though.

THIRD GUEST Your eyes are affected, my lord.

FOURTH GUEST (*to the* FIRST GUEST) I wonder if myopia is brought on by power?

FIRST GUEST (*to the* FOURTH GUEST) I shouldn't have thought so—not necessarily.

SECOND GUEST Oh yes, it happens quite frequently.

As soon as MACBETT *lets go of his throat, the* SERVANT *goes off right.*

MACBETT Perhaps I'm mistaken. (*To the others, who had got up at the same time as he did.*) Sit down, friends. A little wine will clear my head. Anyway, whoever it looks like, Duncan or me, let's smash that picture. Then we'll all have a few drinks. (*He sits down and drinks.*) Why are you looking at me like that? Sit down, I said. We'll all have a few drinks together. (*He stands up and pounds on the table with his fist.*) Sit down!

The GUESTS *sit down.* MACBETT *sits down too.*

Drink, gentlemen, drink. You must admit, I'm a better king than Duncan was.

THIRD GUEST   Hear, hear, my lord!

MACBETT   This country needs a younger man at the helm, braver and more energetic. I can assure you, you haven't lost in the exchange.

FOURTH GUEST   That's what we think, your Highness.

MACBETT   Think! What did you think of Duncan, when he was alive? Did you tell him what you thought? Did you tell him he was the bravest? The most energetic commander? Or did you tell him I should take his place? That I should be king instead of him?

FIRST GUEST   My lord—

MACBETT   I thought he was more suited to it myself. Do you agree? Or do you think differently? Answer me!

SECOND GUEST   My lord—

MACBETT   My lord, my lord, my lord . . . well, what then? You've lost your voice, have you? Anyone who thinks I'm not the best possible ruler, past, present and to come, get up and say so. You don't dare. (*Pause.*) You don't dare. And the greatest. And the most just. You miserable specimens. Go on, get drunk.

The lights go out upstage. The other lot of tables that were projected on the back or reflected by means of mirrors disappear.

BANCO *suddenly appears. When he starts speaking he is framed in the doorway, stage right. He moves forward.*

BANCO   I dare, Macbett.

MACBETT   Banco!

BANCO   I dare tell you you're a traitor, a swindler, and a murderer.

MACBETT (*giving ground*)   You're not dead after all.

The four GUESTS *have risen.* MACBETT *continues to give ground as* BANCO *comes forward.*

Banco! (*He half draws his dagger.*) Banco!

FIRST GUEST (*to* MACBETT)   It's not Banco, my lord.

MACBETT   I tell you it is.

SECOND GUEST   It's not Banco in flesh and blood. It's only his ghost.

MACBETT   His ghost? (*He laughs.*) Yes, it's only a ghost. I can see through it, put my hand through it. So you are dead after all. You don't frighten me. A pity I can't kill you a second time. This is no place for you here.

THIRD GUEST   He's come from Hell.

MACBETT   You've come from Hell and must return. How did you manage it? Show me the pass that Satan's lieutenant gave you. Have you got till midnight? Sit down. In the place of honor. Poor ghost. You can neither eat nor drink. Sit down among my guests here.

The GUESTS *are frightened and draw back.*

What are you worried about? Go up to him. Give him the illusion he exists. He'll despair even more when he returns to his dark abode . . . either too hot or too wet.

BANCO   Scum! All I can do now is curse you.

MACBETT   You can't make me feel any remorse. If I hadn't killed you first, you'd have killed me—as you did Duncan. You struck the first blow, remember? I was going to make you chamberlain, but you wanted to rule in my place.

BANCO   As you took Duncan's place, who made you Baron twice over.

MACBETT (*to the* GUESTS)   There's no cause for alarm. What are you so frightened of? To think I choose my generals from among these crybabies.

BANCO   I trusted you, I followed you, then you and the witches put a spell on me.

MACBETT   You wanted to substitute your progeny for mine. Well, you didn't get very far. All your children, your grandchildren, your great-grandchildren, died in your seed before being born. Why call me names? I just got there first, that's all.

BANCO   You're in for some surprises, Macbett. Make no mistake. You'll pay for this.

MACBETT   He makes me laugh. I say *he:* really all there is are a few odds and ends, the remains of his old personality—leftovers, a robot.

BANCO *disappears.*

At practically the same moment, DUNCAN *appears, mounting the throne.*

FOURTH GUEST   The Archduke! Look, look! The Archduke!

SECOND GUEST   The Archduke!

MACBETT   I'm the only Archduke around here. Look at me, can't you, when you speak to me.

THIRD GUEST   The Archduke! (*He points.*)

MACBETT (*turning*)   Is this some kind of reunion or something?

> *The GUESTS go cautiously up to DUNCAN, but stop a certain distance away. The FIRST and SECOND GUESTS kneel to the right and left of the throne. The two others, further off, are on either side of MACBETT, though a certain distance away.*

> *The three of them, MACBETT and the two GUESTS, have their backs to the audience. The first two are in profile. DUNCAN, on his throne, faces straight out.*

FIRST *and* THIRD GUESTS (*to the* ARCHDUKE)   My lord—

MACBETT   You didn't believe Banco was real, but you seem to believe that Duncan exists all right and is sitting there on the throne. Is it because he was your sovereign that you've grown used to paying him homage and holding him in awe? Now it's my turn to say, "It's only a ghost." (*To* DUNCAN) As you can see, I've taken your throne. And I've taken your wife. All the same, I served you well and you distrusted me. (*To his* GUESTS) Get back to your places. (*He draws his dagger.*) Quickly. You have no king here but me. You pay homage to me now.

> *The GUESTS retreat, terrified.*

And call me "My Lord." Say . . .

GUESTS (*bowing and scraping*)   We hear and obey, my lord. Our happiness is to submit.

FOURTH GUEST   Our greatest happiness is to do what you say.

MACBETT   I see you understand. (*To* DUNCAN) I don't want to see you again till you've been forgiven by the thousands of soldiers I slaughtered in your name, and till they have been pardoned in their turn by the thousands of women that they raped, and by the thousands of children and peasants they killed.

DUNCAN   I've killed or had killed tens of thousands of men and women, soldiers and civilians alike. I've had thousands of homesteads burnt to the ground. True. Very true. But there is one thing that you haven't got quite right. You didn't steal my wife. (*He laughs sardonically.*)

MACBETT   Are you mad? (*To the four* GUESTS) His death has made him balmy—isn't that right, gentlemen?

GUESTS (*one after the other*)   Yes, my lord.

MACBETT (*to* DUNCAN)   Go on, shoo! you silly old ghost.

DUNCAN *disappears behind the throne. He had already stood up to prepare his exit.*

MAID   My lord, my lord! She's disappeared!

MACBETT   Who?

MAID   Your noble wife, my lord. Lady Macbett.

MACBETT   What did you say?

MAID   I went into her room. It was empty. Her things were gone and so was her maid.

MACBETT   Go and find her and bring her to me. She had a headache. She's gone for a walk in the grounds to get a breath of fresh air before coming in to dinner.

MAID We've looked everywhere. We've cried out her name. But only our echoes answered.

MACBETT (*to the four* GUESTS) Scour the forests! Scour the countryside! Bring her to me! (*To the* MAID) Go and look in the attic, in the dungeons, in the cellar. Perhaps she got shut in by mistake. Quickly. Jump to it.

The MAID *goes out.*

And you. Jump to it. Take police dogs. Search every house. Have them close the frontiers. Have patrol boats comb the seas, even outside our territorial waters. Have powerful searchlights sweep the waves. Make contact with our neighboring states to have her expelled and brought back home. If they invoke the right of asylum or say they haven't signed a treaty of extradition, declare war on them. I want reports every quarter of an hour. And arrest all old women who look as if they might be witches. I want all the caves searched.

The MAID *comes in upstage.*

The four GUESTS, *who were feverishly grabbing swords off the wall and buckling them on and getting tangled up in the process, stop suddenly in the midst of all this activity and turn to face the* MAID.

MAID Lady Macbett is coming.

LADY DUNCAN *enters*.

She was just on her way up from the cellar, coming up the stairs. (*The* MAID *goes out.*)

> LADY MACBETT, *or rather* LADY DUNCAN, *is rather different from when she last appeared. She is no longer wearing her crown. Her dress is a bit rumpled.*

FIRST *and* SECOND GUESTS (*together*)   Lady Macbett!

THIRD *and* FOURTH GUESTS (*together*)   Lady Macbett!

FOURTH GUEST   Lady Macbett!

MACBETT   You're rather late, madam. I've turned the whole country upside down, looking for you. Where have you been all this time? I'd like an explanation—but not just now. (*To the four* GUESTS) Sit down, gentlemen. Our wedding feast can now begin. Let's eat, drink, and be merry. (*To* LADY MACBETT) Let's forget our little difference. You've come back, my darling, that's the main thing. Let's feast and enjoy ourselves in the company of our dear friends here, who love you as dearly as I do and who have been waiting eagerly for you to arrive.

> *Upstage the projection or the mirrors with the other* GUESTS *and tables appear again.*

FIRST *and* SECOND GUESTS   Long live Lady Macbett!

THIRD *and* FOURTH GUESTS   Long live Lady Macbett!

MACBETT (*to* LADY MACBETT)   Take the place of honor.

FOURTH GUEST   Lady Macbett, our beloved sovereign!

LADY MACBETT *or* LADY DUNCAN   Beloved or not, I am your sovereign. But I'm not Lady Macbett, I'm Lady Duncan—the unhappy but faithful widow of your rightful king, the Archduke Duncan.

MACBETT (*to* LADY DUNCAN)   Are you mad?

Song. Opera.

FIRST GUEST   She is mad.

SECOND GUEST   Is she mad?

THIRD GUEST   She's off her head.

FOURTH GUEST   She's out of her mind.

FIRST GUEST   We were at her wedding!

MACBETT (*to* LADY DUNCAN)   You're my wife. Surely you can't have forgotten. They were all there at the wedding.

LADY DUNCAN   Not my marriage, no. What you saw was Macbett being married to a sorceress who had taken my face, my voice, my body. She threw me in the palace dungeons and chained me up. Just now my chains fell and the bolts drew back as if by magic. I want nothing to do with you, Macbett. I'm not your accomplice. You murdered your master and your friend. Usurper, imposter.

MACBETT   Then how do you know what's been going on?

FIRST GUEST (*singing*)   Yes, how does she know?

SECOND GUEST (*singing*)   She couldn't have known. She was shut up.

THIRD GUEST (*singing*)   She couldn't have known.

GUESTS (*singing*)   She couldn't have known.

LADY DUNCAN (*speaking*)   I heard all about it on the

prison telegraph. My neighbors tapped out the message on the wall in code. I knew everything there was to know. Well, go and look for her—your beautiful wife, the old hag.

MACBETT (*singing*)   Alas, alas, alas! This time it's not a ghost, it's not a ghost this time.

End of Macbett's sung section.

Yes, I'd like to meet that old hag again. She took the way you look and the way you move and made them still more beautiful. She had a more beautiful voice than yours. Where can I find her? She must have disappeared into mist or into thin air. We have no flying machines to track her down, no devices for tracing unidentified flying objects.

GUESTS (*singing together*)   Long live Macbett, down with Macbett. Long live Macbett, down with Macbett! Long live Lady Duncan, down with Lady Duncan! Long live Lady Duncan, down with Lady Duncan!

LADY DUNCAN (*to* MACBETT)   It doesn't look as if your witch is going to help you any more. Unluckily for you, she's abandoned you.

MACBETT   Unluckily? Aren't I lucky to be king of this country? I don't need anyone's help. (*To the* GUESTS) Get out, you slaves.

They go out.

LADY DUNCAN   You won't get off so lightly. You won't be king for long. Macol, Duncan's son, has just come back from Carthage. He has mustered a large and powerful army. The whole country is against you. You've run out of friends, Macbett. (LADY MACBETT *disappears*.)

Shouts of "Down with Macbett! Long live Macol! Down with Macbett! Long live Macol!"

Fanfares. MACOL *enters.*

MACBETT   I fear no one.

MACOL   So I've found you at last. Lowest of the low, despicable, ignoble, abject creature. Monster, villain, scum, murderer. Moral imbecile. Slimy snake. Acrochord. Horned adder. Foul toad. Filthy slob.

MACBETT   Not very impressive. A foolish boy playing at being an avenger. Psychosomatic cripple. Ridiculous imbecile. Heroic puppy. Infatuated idiot. Presumptuous upstart. Greenhorn ninny.

LADY DUNCAN (*to* MACOL, *indicating* MACBETT)   Kill this unclean man, then throw away your tainted sword.

MACBETT   Silly little sod. Shoo! I killed your fool of a father. I wouldn't like to have to kill you, too. It's no good. You can't hurt me. No man of woman born can harm Macbett.

MACOL   They've pulled the wool over your eyes. They were putting you on.

LADY DUNCAN (*to* MACBETT)   Macol isn't my son. Duncan adopted him. Banco was his father, his mother was a gazelle that a witch transformed into a woman. After bringing Macol into the world, she changed back into a gazelle again. I left the court secretly before he was born so that no one would know that I wasn't pregnant. Everyone took him for my son and Duncan's. He wanted an heir, you see.

MACOL   I shall resume my father's name and found a dynasty that will last for centuries.

LADY DUNCAN   No, Macol. Duncan looked after you. He sent you to Carthage University. You must carry on the family name.

MACBETT   Accursed hags. The most cruelly ironic fate since Oedipus.

MACOL   I'll kill two birds with one stone—revenge both my natural and adoptive fathers. But I won't give up my name.

LADY DUNCAN   Ungrateful boy. You have certain obligations to the memory of Duncan. The whole world is ass-backward. The good behave worse than the bad.

MACOL (*drawing his sword, to* MACBETT)   We have some old scores to settle between us. You're not going to draw your stinking breath one moment longer.

MACBETT   On your own head be it. You're making a bad mistake. I can only be beaten when the forest marches against me.

> MEN *and* WOMEN *approach* MACBETT *and* MACOL *who are center stage. Each of them is carrying a placard with a tree drawn on it—branches would do as well.*
>
> *Recourse should be had to these two solutions only when there are inadequate technical resources. What should really happen is that the whole set, or at least the upstage part of it, should lumber forward to encircle* MACBETT.

MACOL   Look behind you. The forest is on the march.

MACBETT *turns.*

MACBETT   Shit!

MACOL *stabs* MACBETT *in the back.* MACBETT *falls.*

MACOL   Take away this carrion.

Noises off. Shouts of "Long live Macol! Long live Macol! The tyrant is dead! Long live Macol, our beloved sovereign! Long live Macol!"

And bring me a throne.

Two GUESTS *take up Macbett's body. At the same time the throne is brought on.*

GUEST   Please be seated, my lord.

The other GUESTS *arrive. Some of them put up placards reading "Macol is always right."*

GUESTS   Long live Macol! Long live Banco's dynasty! Long live the king!

Sound of bells. MACOL *is by the throne. The* BISHOP *comes on right.*

MACOL (*to the* BISHOP)   You've come to crown me?
BISHOP   Yes, your Highness.

A poor WOMAN *comes on left.*

WOMAN   May your reign be a happy one!

SECOND WOMAN (*coming on right*)   Spare a thought for the poor!

MAN (*coming on right*)   No more injustice.

SECOND MAN   Hate has destroyed our house. Hate has poisoned our souls.

THIRD MAN   May your reign usher in a time of peace, harmony and concord.

FIRST WOMAN   May your reign be blessed.

SECOND WOMAN   A time of joy.

MAN   A time of love.

ANOTHER MAN   Let us embrace, my brothers.

BISHOP   And I will give you my blessing.

MACOL (*standing in front of the throne*)   Silence!

FIRST WOMAN   He's going to speak.

FIRST MAN   The king is going to speak.

SECOND WOMAN   Let's listen to what he has to say.

SECOND MAN   We're listening, my lord. We'll drink your words.

ANOTHER MAN   God bless you.

BISHOP   God bless you.

MACOL   Quiet, I say. Don't all talk at once. I'm going to make an announcement. Nobody move. Nobody breathe. Now get this into your heads. Our country sank beneath the yoke, each day a new gash was added to her wounds. But I have trod upon the tyrant's head and now wear it on my sword.

A MAN *comes on with Macbett's head on the end of a pike.*

THIRD MAN   You got what was coming to you.

SECOND WOMAN   He got what was coming to him.

FOURTH MAN   I hope God doesn't forgive him.

FIRST WOMAN   Let him be damned eternally.

FIRST MAN   Let him burn in Hell.

SECOND MAN   I hope they torture him.

THIRD MAN   I hope he doesn't get a moment's peace.

FOURTH MAN   I hope he repents in the flames and God refuses him.

FIRST WOMAN   I hope they tear his tongue out and it grows again, and they pull it out again twenty times a day.

SECOND MAN   I hope they roast him on a spit. I hope they impale him. I hope he can see how happy we are. I hope our laughter deafens him.

SECOND WOMAN   I've got my knitting needles. Let's put his eyes out.

MACOL   If you don't shut up at once, I'll set my soldiers and dogs on you.

A forest of guillotines appears upstage as in the First Scene.

MACOL   Now that the tyrant is dead and curses his mother for bringing him into the world, I'll tell you this: My poor country shall have more vices than it had before, more suffer and more sundry ways than ever by me that do succeed.

As Macol's announcement continues, there are murmurs of discontent, amazement and despair from the crowd. At the end of the speech, MACOL is left alone.

EUGÈNE IONESCO

In me I know
All the particulars of vice so grafted
That, when they shall be opened, black
Macbett will seem as pure as snow and the
   poor state
Esteem him as a lamb, being compared
With my confineless harms. I grant him bloody.
Luxurious, avaricious, false, deceitful,
Sudden, malicious, smacking of every sin
That has a name: but there's no bottom, none,
In my voluptuousness. Your wives, your daughters,
Your matrons, and your maids, cannot fill up
The cistern of my lust, and my desire
All continent impediments shall o'erbear
That do oppose my will. Better Macbett,
Than such a one to reign. With this there grows
In my most ill-composed affection, such
a staunchless avarice, that now I'm king
I shall cut off the nobles from their lands,
Desire his jewels, and this other's house,
And my more-having will be as a sauce
To make my hunger more, that I shall forge
Quarrels unjust against the good and loyal,
Destroying them for wealth. The king—
   becoming graces
As justice, verity, temp'rance, stableness,
Bounty, perseverance, mercy, lowliness.
Devotion, patience, courage, fortitude,
I have no relish of them, but abound
In the division of each several crime,
Acting it many ways.

The BISHOP, *who was the only one left, goes de-jectedly out right.*

Now I have power, I shall
Pour the sweet milk of concord into Hell,
Uproar the universal peace, confound
All unity on earth.
First I'll make this Archduchy a kingdom—
and me the king. An empire—and me the
emperor. Super-highness, super-king,
super-majesty, emperor of emperors.

He disappears in the mist.

The mist clears. The BUTTERFLY HUNTER *crosses the stage.*